Beyond Banting

Beyond Banting

From Insulin to Islet Transplants,
Decoding Canada's Diabetes Research Superstars

Krista Lamb

Rock's Mills Press
Oakville, Ontario
2021

Published by
Rock's Mills Press
www.rocksmillspress.com

*For Donald, who always knew I had a book in me,
and Shawn, who helped me bring this one into the world.*

Contents

Author's Note

Some of the interviews in this book originally aired on the *Diabetes Canada Podcast*, of which I am the producer and host. I am incredibly grateful to Diabetes Canada for allowing me to reproduce some of that content. Many of the research programs featured in this book were funded by Diabetes Canada, which has provided millions of dollars to support projects that further improve education, treatment, and the search for a cure.

You can find the *Diabetes Canada Podcast* on all the usual channels or by visiting diabetes.ca/resources/podcast.

Foreword

Dr. Jan Hux

Past President and CEO, Diabetes Canada

In my role as Chief Science Officer at Diabetes Canada, I was often approached by staff from the communications team with requests to help them tell the story of the research and researchers that the organization funded. So, I was not surprised when a newly hired communications manager named Krista Lamb landed in my office and asked me to "tell her about research." Krista's previous employment had been in the entertainment and social services sectors so she came to the role with good communications skills but very little relevant content expertise. I'm afraid I wasn't optimistic.

However, over the subsequent months and years, I was amazed to observe her genuine and growing interest in the subject and her willingness to engage with fields of research as disparate as foundational biomedical studies and glucose management in high-performance athletes. She had no aspiration to become a researcher herself, yet she had clearly been bitten by the research bug. This book is the fruit of that newly discovered passion.

Diabetes is inherently a story of both science and people. The processes that control the metabolism of the food we eat are complex and made more complex still when, through the impact of a range of genetic and environmental factors, diabetes interferes with them. What is taught in Grade 10 science as a simple sequence of digestion of food and absorption of nutrients, turns out to be far more intricate with local cells in the intestinal wall and pancreas operating under the influence of factors ranging from neurons in the brain to bacteria living in the gut.

But it is also a human story. The people living with diabetes need to learn, often from an early age in the case of type 1 diabetes, how to pinch hit for a pancreas that has stopped reliably delivering the right amount of lifesaving insulin. It is a task that has obvious medical implications but also far-reaching social and psychological impacts on those affected by it. Those human stories, stories of heroic achievement and heartbreaking losses that I heard in my time as a clinician and as an advocate, have left a lasting mark on me as they do on all who work in the diabetes field.

In this lively and engaging volume, Krista has captured both the science of diabetes research in Canada and the human stories of the people who have dedicated their lives to solving its mysteries. In some cases, the trajectory is from bench to bedside, as for Dan Drucker, whose deep immersion into the biology of incretins culminated in the development of two new classes of drugs to manage type 2 diabetes. In other cases, the plot gets unravelled from the other end, prompted by a patient's story that doesn't fit the existing science. This was the case in Heather Dean's identification of youth onset type 2 diabetes in First Nations communities and the work of the team she inspired to get to the root of the biology (and history and sociology) behind the unexpected finding.

In 2021, Canadians will be rightly proud to celebrate the 100th anniversary of the discovery of insulin. As the Nobel committee noted when announcing the award to Banting and MacLeod, it was a discovery of great theoretical and practical significance. But we do not need to look back nearly that far to find Canadian diabetes researchers who are pushing the theoretical boundaries of the relevant physiology, pathology, genetics and immunology. Nor do we need to reach back a century to find Canadians who are generating innovations of great practical significance for the lives of those affected by diabetes. At academic medical facilities all across the country, exciting advances in diabetes research are being pursued, and Canada continues to punch above its weight in this important field. The book you are about to read, of necessity, profiles only a selected few stories, but surely enough to stoke the pride of Canadians and fuel our anticipation of more life-transforming discoveries in the years to come.

Beyond Banting

Diabetes and Me

Diabetes entered the periphery of my life at an early age. A boy in my class named Darryl had it. This is one of the things I remember most clearly from elementary school. While the rest of us lived a typical 1980s childhood, fueled by a diet of Fruit Roll-Ups and those little packets of Cheez-Whiz with white crackers, Darryl had a special eating regimen because he had diabetes.

I didn't really get it then. I just knew that Darryl was adorable and that he made the heart of this second grader beat faster whenever he was around. But I don't remember thinking much about his diabetes. In my eyes, it was like being the kid with braces or glasses, or whatever other small difference many of us had to deal with. Only it wasn't. I get that now. But in typical little-kid fashion, I just understood that he was special because he needed to be treated a little differently.

My grandmothers also both had diabetes. This means I'm much more likely to develop it myself. Their diabetes was different than Darryl's though, something I didn't really understand as I was growing up. Darryl had what would have then been termed "Juvenile Diabetes" (it's now called type 1 diabetes). It's thought to be an autoimmune disease wherein the pancreas no longer produces the insulin the body needs to function. It happens most frequently in children and young adults—hence the "juvenile" part—though, in recent years, it has begun to be diagnosed more frequently in adults.

I know all of these things because diabetes has followed me since my school days with Darryl. My first crush on a little boy with type 1 diabetes didn't really register as overly important at the time, but now I wonder if it was the universe's way of setting me on a path, one where I would encounter and discover much more about the disease. The diabetes both my grandmothers had was type 2, the one most commonly associated with lifestyle—though it's actually a complex combination of things like genetics, socioeconomic status, and the area where you live. It's much more complicated than just diet and exercise. In many ways, my grandmothers' experiences with the condition resonated more strongly with me because they were family.

Growing up, my Grandmother Lamb came to stay with us for a few months when I was around seven or eight. My mother told me later that her mother-in-law was supposed to stay a few weeks at most, but once she was fully ensconced in my childhood bedroom in my parents' basement, she showed no signs of leaving. This made life much more difficult for my mother, who was now forced to shuffle the sleeping arrangements of two young children in our too-small bungalow. She also had to manage my grandmother's special diet, and like many women, my mother had a complicated relationship with her mother-in-law.

My grandmother smoked too much. She was also stately and demanding, and did not suffer fools gladly. She was a woman who'd raised five sons in a remote area of Nova Scotia, and by the time my brother and I came along, the by-products of my father's later-in-life second marriage, she was already a very set-in-her-ways person.

Today, I don't know that *I* could handle having her as a mother-in-law, but as a grandmother, she was the best. I remember dancing with her in our living room, sitting next to her while she read one of the romance novels she owned in an astonishing quantity, and keeping her company every night as she ate the second dinner my mother begrudgingly prepared for her: Corn Flakes and toast with butter. It was a terrible onslaught of carbs in retrospect, but now I assume it was meant to keep her blood sugar up throughout the night. Hypoglycemia may also have been responsible for my grandmother's moodiness, which my mother remembers in vivid detail, but in those days, these connections between emotions and the body weren't quite so well understood. My grandmother was rail thin, and other than her advanced age, she wasn't someone who you'd think—given the stereotypes—would have diabetes.

My Grandma Barter, on the other hand, was pleasantly plump and inordinately good natured. She lived in rural Québec and was the quintessential grandmother—always happy to have you in her kitchen as she baked cookies. She was the polar opposite of my Grandmother Lamb in every way. She had none of her elegance, but she was filled with joy. Whereas Grandmother Lamb always seemed a bit distant, Grandma Barter was full of laughter and hugs.

It wasn't at all unusual that Grandma Barter had developed type 2 diabetes. She carried a bit too much weight, she loved sweets, and it ran in her family. She was also afflicted with heart disease, which is equally prevalent on my mother's side. Since Grandma Barter and I are very much alike in build and temperament, it makes me worry about my own potential risk in developing these diseases, as I know all too well that genetics plays almost as much of a role as lifestyle in type 2 diabetes risk (not that you'd learn that by watching news reports on diabetes).

I grew up visiting my mother's family every summer, and as I watched my grandma check her blood sugar throughout the day, it didn't faze me. She was always pulling out her test kit and needles as we sat around her big kitchen table. She did her best, but she couldn't resist a night out at the only Chinese restaurant in town or eating a cookie after her meal. She tried hard, but she loved life and food and all the good things we associate with being fully alive. I don't begrudge her any of that.

Diabetes was a big part of my childhood, and it continued to lurk in the background during my teenage years. When I grew out of elementary school boys, my first rock star crush (and this is painful to admit) was Bret Michaels, the lead singer of the glam rock band, Poison. I was smitten with the pretty blond man wearing too much makeup, who often favoured multiple scarves wrapped around his neck.

I was aware that Michaels had type 1 diabetes, which probably made it more difficult for him to live the sex, drugs, and rock 'n' roll lifestyle. But, just as with Darryl and my grandmothers, I sort of glossed over this fact. All I knew was that this was the man whose poster I wanted taped to my bedroom ceiling, despite my father's protests. He was adamant that the tape would leave a mark, and it did.

After graduation, I studied journalism and then moved into working in entertainment communications. I loved telling the stories of the musicians I represented. When George Canyon became a client at our agency, he had not yet become one of Canada's most well-known country music performers. We started working with him before his second-place finish on the televised music competition *Nashville Star* and the fame that followed that achievement. To me, the fact that he had type 1 diabetes seemed nothing more than an interesting footnote.

Canyon often told the story of how his dream of becoming an air force pilot was sidelined by his diabetes diagnosis at the age of thirteen. He was a big, strapping cowboy with a square jaw, and he seemed to be the picture of health. I don't think I truly understood what it must have been like for Canyon to realize that a disease that was in no way his fault had robbed him of his childhood dream.

I look back now and regret the lack of empathy I had for him. He worked a gruelling schedule on the road those first few years. We booked him on morning television and breakfast radio shows, even on days when he'd been performing the night before, as these were the things he had to do to sell albums and concert tickets—as well as keep his songs on the radio. This is hard enough on its own, let alone while trying to manage an incredibly complex disease that involves constant vigilance.

For those with type 1 diabetes, every meal has to be carefully considered, every carb counted. Any type of exercise and activity can lead to swings in blood sugar that are often difficult to predict and get a handle on. Going from life at home to life on the road, where you never quite know what food will be available, plus putting on shows every night and doing endless rounds of media on little to no sleep— it's a wonder he held it together at all.

But as I've gotten to know many more people living with type 1 diabetes over the years, I've discovered that they are also incredibly resilient. These days, George Canyon's diabetes is so well-managed that he has been awarded a commercial pilot's licence and is now able to fly with passengers—a right he fought hard to earn, both for himself and the many other people with type 1 diabetes who hoped to become pilots. He has spent years as an advocate for JDRF (formerly the Juvenile Diabetes Research Foundation) and other diabetes-related charities, meeting with thousands of children who live with type 1 diabetes and assuring them that the diagnosis does not have to stop them from chasing down their own dreams.

I stopped working with Canyon in 2007, but my work in diabetes hasn't abated. In 2014, I took on the role of Communications Manager for Diabetes Canada (then called the Canadian Diabetes Association). I had been interested in medical research for many years, and I liked the idea of telling the stories of those affected by this disease—as well as the researchers trying to cure it.

Little did I know then that I had found my calling. At Diabetes Canada, I met so many people living with the condition or affected by it. I also encountered health care providers who were on the frontlines of research and care. I learned about the day-to-day struggles of those with type 1 and those who had developed type 2 diabetes. I met children who were diagnosed before they could even walk, as well as adults who had no risk factors, and yet still developed type 2 diabetes based on a cruel twist of genetics. I learned about the incredible financial burdens of this illness, too, and about the stigma those living with the condition face. We've come a long way in how we treat and describe this disease—but we still have much farther to go.

I also met the researchers who are working on treatments to cure the disease. My colleagues and I visited Banting House in London, Ontario, where Sir Frederick Banting woke up from a dream on October 31, 1920, with an idea he felt might just hold the answer to treating diabetes. His middle-of-the-night epiphany led to the discovery of insulin, and it became a treatment that turned a diabetes diagnosis from a death sentence to a more manageable disease.

Insulin may not be a cure, and it's definitely not an easy treatment to navigate, but it's better than dying the way many people needlessly did before the discovery. As I watched my colleagues and friends take a moment to sit on the very bed where Banting had his aha moment, it was hard not to be swept up in the emotion and pride of what he had achieved. Without insulin, so many of the people in my life who have inspired me, loved me, mentored me, and supported me would not be here.

Canada's contribution to diabetes treatment is incredible, but as I went about my work at Diabetes Canada, I was surprised by how little people knew about the research that continues to be done here, in labs across our country. These researchers are continuing Banting's legacy in the hopes of bringing us closer to an elusive cure that would be life-changing for those who live with the disease.

Much of society views diabetes the way I did growing up. Something that the elderly develop. Something not that serious. Something you can manage with just a pill or an injection. Next to cancer or ALS or any of the other devastating diseases out there, it doesn't seem like that big of a deal. My time at Diabetes Canada, however, changed my original perception completely.

There are no vacations from diabetes. People who develop the condition must manage it day in and day out, every day. For young people that are diagnosed in childhood, this means that their parents must be constantly vigilant. It is a life filled with never-ending monitoring to ensure their child's blood sugars do not go too high or too low. Parents also have to confirm that their children take the right dosages of insulin to manage the food that they consume and the activities they take part in.

Much of it is guesswork—what raised your blood sugar on Monday may not do the same on Tuesday—and it is incredibly complicated to try and figure it all out. But these parents do it because they want their children to be healthy and avoid the potentially devastating complications that can come with the disease, like blindness or amputation. Above all, these parents put in the work every day because none of them wants to wake up one morning to find out their child did not make it through the night.

This is a reality of diabetes that we don't talk about—this all-encompassing fear. And it's not just parents who are raising children with the disease who feel this on a daily basis. It's the people living with it, as well. It's a revelation that made me re-evaluate everything I knew about the illness.

Remember Darryl, that adorable little boy in my grade school class? I recall his mom being there at birthday parties and thinking it was a bit strange. But of course she was—she had to count carbs and check his blood sugars. People with diabetes can eat the same things as anyone else, but they have to manage how it impacts their blood glucose to ensure there isn't too much of a high or a low. Every day that Darryl's mom sent him off to school, she must have been wondering if he would be OK. If the teacher would help him if he wasn't. If someone could administer glucagon, a hormone that quickly raises blood sugar levels, if he developed hypoglycemia (a battle that continues with school boards in many provinces, despite the life-or-death consequences).

When Darryl went to high school, he probably faced the stigma and confusion that comes along with being different. While elementary school students can be cruel, it's nothing compared to high school. I didn't know him then, but I wonder how I would have looked at a teenage boy with diabetes. Many young people with type 1 talk about this, the "otherness" that comes with the condition. They are often the only ones in their school with diabetes, and like any typical teenager, they tend to shy away from being different in any way. This makes them less likely to test as much as needed, and less likely to follow the very strict management process they need in order to stay healthy. Unfortunately, this behaviour often makes them much more susceptible to devastating diabetes complications in adulthood.

* * * * *

It was during my time working at Diabetes Canada that all the pieces of the diabetes puzzle fell into place for me. I began to understand in a new way the realities of a life with diabetes. While you can never truly understand a condition you don't live with, as I met more and more people living with diabetes and spoke with them about their experiences, I found myself increasingly drawn to finding ways I could help. This was also when I discovered just how much the Canadian research community is doing to try to improve treatments.

I want people to know the real difference Canadian researchers are continuing to make in the fight against diabetes, and that it did not simply end with Sir Frederick Banting. Every day, across this country, researchers in labs from coast to coast are moving us ever closer to a cure.

Dr. Bruce Perkins, a leading expert on the complications of diabetes who himself lives with type 1 diabetes, was the first researcher who appeared on the *Diabetes Canada Podcast* when it launched in 2017, and his early involvement encouraged other researchers to take a chance and be on the show. The episodes are twenty minutes or less, which I think is the perfect amount of time for a diabetes podcast, but when I'm at a party telling someone about the role of Alberta's research community on developing islet transplants (yes, I'm that person—you don't have to invite me over), I know there's so much more to the story that I still want to share. And that's why I'm doing this.

The podcast initially gave me a platform to start telling these stories, and this book gives me the chance to contribute even more. A book about medical research is hard to write, however, because, like most research, it's tremendously complicated. There are many of you who are probably wondering what the heck an islet is right now—believe me, I've been there, and I'll get to it.

Medical research moves incredibly slowly (just ask anyone who is watching a potential treatment enter phase-three clinical trials years after it was first announced), but medical breakthroughs can also come about quickly. So maybe you're reading this thinking, why should I care about something that still isn't approved, or might never work, or hasn't yet cured this disease after all this time?

Well, because we didn't discover insulin without a lot of time and dedication on the part of Banting and his co-discoverers, Charles Best, James Collip, and John Macleod. We also didn't discover stem cells without making a lot of mistakes along the way. And the stories of the people who dedicate their lives to this work are what make it all worthwhile. I may have spent ten years working in the music industry, but the real rock stars in my life are right here on these pages.

This book is not an exhaustive study of every great research accomplishment in Canada since the time of Banting, Best, Collip, and Macleod. There are so many other talented researchers who have made enormous contributions that I could have written about, but that would make up a whole other book.

There is Dr. Pere Santamaria, who came from Spain to the University of Alberta in 1992 with a goal of studying autoimmune disorders like type 1 diabetes. Arriving with his wife and young child, he discovered that there was no funding for his position, and he had to scrape together the resources to continue his work in nanoparticles. With the help of Diabetes Canada, he was able to start his research program. Now, as he works on a way to reset autoimmune disorders when they first start to appear, he is quietly surpassing all the goals he's set.

Dr. Hertzel Gerstein is another example. He is larger than life. He has no indoor voice, and his enthusiasm is so big it seems to burst out of his small frame. When he asked his entire department at Hamilton Health Sciences to film a video of his diabetes-themed song—an inspiring anthem about overcoming adversity—they were on board. Gerstein, with his head of grey hair and oversize lab coat, sports sunglasses and raps midway through the song. That the man with hip-hop in his heart is also credited with coining the term dysglycemia and has led numerous international clinical trials is perhaps more of a shock.

Reversing type 2 diabetes is one of those things researchers have spent decades working on, with little to show for the effort. Dr. Ravi Retnakaran has actually started to see some promise in his plan to use large doses of insulin at first diagnosis to reverse the disease. Will his quiet, unassuming voice and his potential cure slip under the radar in a field full of those more likely to shout their results?

Dr. Stewart Harris, Dr. Tony Hanley and Dr. Bernard Zinman

have worked with the community in Sandy Lake, Ontario for decades to develop a collaborative process to try and stem the overwhelming epidemic of type 2 diabetes in this Indigenous community. It is a project that has changed hearts and minds and made a real difference.

And Toronto's Dr. Patricia Brubaker has become one of the world's leading experts on GLP agonists. Her work has led to breakthroughs that are shaping how diabetes and other conditions are being treated.

Truly, I could have written a hundred more chapters and never told all the diabetes research success stories coming out of Canada. My main goal is to introduce a larger audience to just a few of the scientists whose stories have inspired me, and the projects I find fascinating and compelling. I hope these stories will motivate others—perhaps the next generation of Canadian research superstars—to expand and further this country's scientific legacy.

No one in this book has cured diabetes—yet. And maybe they never will, but they are doing *so* much to further our understanding of the disease, improve treatments, and bring us ever closer to that moment when no parent will look at their newly diagnosed child with type 1 diabetes and worry that they won't make it through the night. I firmly believe that Canada will be at the forefront of the next diabetes research breakthrough, and after meeting all the people profiled in this book, I think you will, too.

CHAPTER ONE
Basic Science with Big Impact

Dr. Daniel J. Drucker does not like scientists who overstate their findings. He rolls his eyes at media headlines that tout a cure when that's not the case. He is also the first to call someone out on Twitter when they've made a claim that doesn't hold up. He gets frustrated when funding is allocated to science just because it sounds exciting, even when the work behind it isn't sound. He is annoyed by conferences that don't bring in female scientists to speak. He is aggrieved by the lack of buy-in for funding new treatments despite solid evidence that the results will truly help patients.

No one is a bigger advocate for research than Drucker, but he's grown exhausted by the hype and the continued barriers. This creates a slight challenge in writing about him because he's arguably the Canadian who has had the greatest impact on diabetes treatment since Sir Frederick Banting discovered insulin in 1921.

While Banting's name is emblazoned on buildings, stamps, and scholarships, Drucker's is far less recognizable outside of the scientific community. But if you are diagnosed with type 2 diabetes, there is a good chance you will one day be prescribed a GLP-1 agonist, one of the medications Drucker's research has made possible. The Montréal-born scientist may not have his name on a statue, and perhaps he'd really hate it if he did, but his contribution to diabetes treatment and care is nothing short of remarkable.

Those who work with Drucker are less unassuming about what

he has accomplished. "We should all recognize that his research has led to three different classes of medications used in diabetes, and in other conditions," says Toronto's Dr. Bruce Perkins, a clinician-scientist, and the director of Mount Sinai's Leadership Sinai Centre for Diabetes. "No one accomplishes this in a career. It's phenomenal. These drugs have changed diabetes management and are extremely effective medications for type 2 diabetes."

There are millions of scientists working around the world at any given time, and few will experience a breakthrough that is remarkable enough to have a lasting impact on health care in their lifetime. Dan Drucker has had *three*. To put it into a more understandable context, Drucker is to diabetes research what Tom Brady is to football.

This is all on my mind the first time I meet Drucker in his office at Mount Sinai Hospital, to interview him about his upcoming keynote talk at the Diabetes Canada/Canadian Society of Endocrinology and Metabolism Professional Conference. There, he would be giving a presentation about his discovery of the important role GLP-1 agonists play in treating type 2 diabetes.

I am not a scientist. This fact was important as I prepared for my interview with Drucker and will likely be even more important to understand as you read this book. I did not even take any science classes past high school. The only one I'd really had an interest in was environmental science, in which my class trekked off to Toronto's High Park to test the pH levels in Grenadier Pond, allowing us to experience something that seemed more important than what was found in textbooks. I had boycotted the frog dissection in grade 10 biology and basically scoffed at the idea of taking chemistry or physics. After all, I was going to be a *journalist*—not a scientist.

And yet, as an adult, I've grown to love science—medical research in particular. All the information in the textbooks seems far more pressing through an adult lens. I recognize and admire all the brilliant minds who are taking our understanding of medical science to a different level in the hopes of preventing or treating diseases.

Now, I was waiting for the elevator to take me to the office of one of the world's preeminent diabetes researchers, silently mouthing the proper pronunciation of "incretin" over and over again. While I can more than hold my own in conversations with scientists these days, there was still something about meeting Drucker, who has a reputation for being, shall we say, *intense,* that had me wanting to bring my A-game. I most definitely wanted to say the name of the type of hormones he'd built his career on correctly.

Drucker's office at the Lunenfeld-Tanenbaum Research Institute in Toronto, where he is a senior scientist, is sparsely decorated. When he stands to greet me, I am immediately thrown by how small he seems in comparison to the weight of his reputation. Wearing slim-fitting green pants with a white polo-style shirt, he gives off a relaxed and casual air.

His raspy voice can come across as gruff when you first meet him, and I suspect he brooks no fools, but he also strikes me as remarkably warm. In his early sixties, he does not look his age, though a telling mention of his grandkids and a quick calculation of his career gives it away.

Speaking with him that day, I realize that while he may be a larger-than-life presence, he is also patient and helpful—happy to take the time to break down the incredibly complex science he works on for a lay audience. He doesn't even flinch when I invariably butcher "incretin" during our conversation. He is affable and friendly, despite the weariness in his voice when he talks about the state of science funding today.

He has earned the right to be outspoken on this topic, as without the funding and support his lab has received over his more than thirty-year career, none of his accomplishments would be possible. It also concerns him that without further investment, the next generation of scientists are being set up to fail. The odds are already against them and taking away funding simply widens that gap.

Just as Sir Frederick Banting never set out to study diabetes, Dan Drucker had no intention of working in this field at all. Arriving at Dr. Joel Habener's lab at Massachusetts General Hospital in Boston in 1984, he had studied medicine at the University of Toronto and was determined to work in thyroid research. That goal was sidelined when there were no spots left in the program, and instead, he found himself assigned to study the glucagon gene.

"It was very unplanned, very serendipitous," he says now, a hint of a shrug in his gravelly voice. "I still kept up my interest in thyroid disease, but I spent the majority of my research career trying to understand gut peptides and obesity in diabetes."

A missed opportunity for him turned out to be a boon for those diagnosed with type 2 diabetes. Drucker's work is called basic science, meaning it's at the foundational or discovery level. This is the fundamental research done to better understand how things work. This type of preclinical research typically does not make for big headlines. His work involves asking intricate questions, then setting out to answer them methodically, understanding that he may be wrong far more often than he is right.

Type 2 diabetes is the more prevalent of the two forms of the disease. It is also the one most often associated with lifestyle, though it turns out to be far more complicated than that. Diabetes Canada estimates there are more than 11 million people in the country who live with diabetes or prediabetes (when blood sugar levels are elevated but not high enough to be diagnosed as type 2 diabetes). Of those, more than 90 percent are living with prediabetes or type 2 diabetes—type 1 diabetes still remains relatively rare in comparison.

The reasons for this epidemic are complex. "We know that lifestyle plays a role, but it goes far beyond that," says Dr. Jan Hux, retired president and CEO of Diabetes Canada. "Ethnicity, genetic predisposition, the built environment, food insecurity—all of these and so much more come into play when you look at why a person is at risk."

Basic scientists in the diabetes field look at what is happening in our bodies to try and understand the intricate mechanisms that determine why and how diabetes develops. They then try to figure out why, for example, one person who is obese develops type 2 diabetes while another person who is also obese does not. Why a slender and active person is diagnosed when someone who is overweight and sedentary isn't. In the lab, these scientists study animal models of the disease, searching for triggers and clues that will solve these complex puzzles.

It is often thankless work, as much of the glory in research goes to the clinicians who take the work of basic scientists and craft it into treatments and cures. It is also extremely time-intensive and fraught with scientific failure. Often, scientists spend decades working on something that only leads to an incremental understanding of an issue. That initial work can be pivotal for future scientists, however, who take that kernel of knowledge even further.

Such was the case for Drucker. The role of glucagon-like peptides in diabetes and obesity has been explored for decades in labs all over the world. Starting in the 1970s, researchers began to see the potential of gut peptides, and in 1984, Drucker applied what had been learned in the preceding decade with the cloning of the glucagon gene and began his own experiments. During the years that followed, he made remarkable progress, but the wheels of medical science turn very slowly.

While Banting and his co-discoverers of insulin may have been able to have their breakthrough in the summer and begin human testing in the fall, these days, safety and careful consideration have slowed the process down considerably. Once a theory has been shown to be viable, it must go through extensive testing in animal models before it can be tested in humans. If these trials are successful, they are approved by the applicable governing bodies and made available for the average patient. For example, it was 2005 before a treatment based on Drucker's findings was available to the public.

This dogged pursuit of something worth researching is an essential trait in a scientist. Even if you are just putting together the links that pave the way for the future scientist who finally makes the celebrated breakthrough, the discovery-level work is still essential.

Since the science Drucker does is extremely complex, let's break it down into more easily digestible pieces. First, you need to understand that GLP-1, which stands for glucagon-like peptide 1, is a naturally occurring hormone, also called an incretin, that all humans make. When we eat, our bodies secrete GLP-1 from our gut endocrine cells, and this incretin stimulates insulin and inhibits glucagon, as well as controlling appetite.

In studying GLP-1, Drucker and his team noted that these same properties would work well as a diabetes drug. GLP-1, he explains, does all this in a glucose-dependent mechanism of action. If you give someone a glucose-lowering drug, it doesn't stop working when their glucose returns to normal. This can lead to hypoglycemia, or extremely low blood sugar, in some patients. With GLP-1, you could lower glucose, but also have the process stop once the normal range has been achieved. For someone with diabetes who experiences regular hypoglycemia, this can be transformative.

The fascinating thing about basic science is that it doesn't always start out with lofty—or even specific—goals. "We never really set out to discover anything. I think, like most scientists, we were just trying to figure out how mechanisms worked," he explains. "Through a series of very small, incremental studies, none of which were flashy and most of which were not published in exciting journals with eye-catching titles, our group and many others in Canada, along with the United States and Europe, gradually began to piece together how these peptides and their control mechanisms worked."

This matter-of-factness is typical of Drucker's style. What he achieved with GLP-1 was ground-breaking, and the medicines that were developed from his basic research (GLP-1 receptor agonists) have had an enormous impact on people living with type 2 diabetes. They have been especially beneficial to those who have not responded well to treatment with sulfonylureas drugs, which are used to increase insulin production and are often prescribed alongside metformin—the first-line therapy most type 2 diabetes patients receive.

He is equally pragmatic about his second major discovery. Scientists at the University of British Columbia (UBC), including Dr. John Brown, and later Drs. Ray Pederson and Chris McIntosh, established a leading program in gut hormones and the biology of DPP-4, the enzyme that breaks down many gut hormones.

Drucker, building on this work and other studies from the University of Copenhagen, demonstrated that if you prevent DPP-4 (the enzyme that breaks down GLP-1) from working, GLP-1 lasts longer and lowers glucose. This work led to another class of medications—

DPP-4 inhibitors—which are currently helping people better manage their type 2 diabetes. DPP-4 inhibitors are often prescribed after metformin has been tried for the management of type 2 diabetes. These medicines are popular as they are generally well tolerated, though they remain prohibitively expensive for many.

Medications based on Drucker's work are now so ubiquitous that even his late mother-in-law was once prescribed one of these drugs. Originally put on a sulfonylureas glucose-lowering drug, she was beset with terrible hypoglycemia. Once she was switched to a DPP-4 inhibitor, which prevented her blood sugar from dipping too low, her life was transformed. I can only imagine this put her son-in-law in her good graces.

A third discovery made by Drucker and Toronto's Dr. Patricia Brubaker has helped develop a treatment for short bowel syndrome, a rare condition where a person does not have enough small intestine and, therefore, their body cannot absorb enough nutrients. This further solidified Drucker's status as one of the world's premier research scientists.

Still, he notes, all his work came about because of basic science, not the stuff that typically gets much attention in the media—or even in scientific journals. "Nothing that you would be excited about, nothing that you would want to throw millions of dollars at, just good old basic science and serendipity. If you support basic science, you'll likely garner unexpected dividends. Whereas if you target big science with grandiose ambitions, you may or may not get the dividends you expected."

Drucker's prolific accomplishments are due in part to his precise and agile scientific mind, but his dogged determination and insistence on excellence are just as important. His oldest son, Aaron, now a clinician-scientist himself, remembers spending time with his dad in the basement laboratories at Toronto General Hospital growing up.

He always knew his parents were physicians and scientists (his mother, Cheryl, is one of the country's leading dermatologists) and that his father was driven to succeed. Drucker expected the same dedication in his children. Yet, Drucker still took time to coach their sports teams, attend their games, and nurture their talents. "He wasn't a crazy hockey parent or anything like that," his son Aaron notes, "But he wanted us to try hard at everything that we did."

Dr. Erin Mulvihill, now a scientist at the University of Ottawa Heart Institute, was drawn to that same quality in Drucker when she became a part of his lab in 2011 as a postdoctoral student. "Research excellence," she says of what motivated her decision to apply for a role in his lab, noting that it's one of the best in the country. She was also impressed with the fact that, unlike many basic research labs, Drucker's was having a real impact on patients—something she could tell truly mattered to him. "Not all science is like that, where people really care about doing basic science that's important to patients. But for Dan, that's his number one motivating factor. If it's not going to help people, then he doesn't want to invest a lot of time researching it."

Part of this drive comes from the years Drucker spent as a physician. He gave up his clinical practice long ago in order to focus on research, but it's clear his patients remain on his mind. He notes that he still talks to many on the phone, and his son, Aaron, is often surprised by how much his dad's impact as a doctor is felt.

"He still has patients coming up to him in the grocery store, and he hasn't practiced medicine for ten years." To the younger Drucker, this is an important reminder for all clinician-scientists, who often get wrapped up in their research and lose sight of the people living with the diseases they seek to treat. "Even if you have a career that focuses on research, make sure you spend the appropriate amount of time with your patients and treat your patients well. It's critically important because first and foremost, you're a physician."

These lessons about remembering the people who your science aims to treat are also important when thinking about the people you are training to become the next generation of great scientists. With a career spanning more than three decades, Drucker has seen dozens of young scientists come through his lab. "I'm an old guy now," he says with a chuckle, though he is only in his sixties, noting that some of his original trainees are now heading toward retirement.

Drucker is known for seeking out excellence and spending time looking for those best suited to answer the specific questions he is hoping to work on at that moment. While he has a reputation for being brusque at times, each of his former lab members I speak with tells me his team is an exceptional place to learn—and one they found to be surprisingly nurturing of their talent.

Drucker is incredibly invested in the outcomes and output of his staff. While he does not meddle or micromanage, his is the sort of lab where you get out as much as you put in. He does not raise his voice or push his trainees to perform. He simply sets them up for success as best he can and then lets them run with it. Or not.

For Dr. Erin Mulvihill, this was an extraordinary opportunity to learn. In Drucker's lab, which is well-funded and staffed, she had access to anything she could possibly need to succeed in her experiments. She also had a mentor who was incredibly driven and happy to provide whatever support he could if he thought her idea was a good one—often at breakneck speed.

"He doesn't put things off. If it can be done, it will be done," she says. "And when you're excited about the work, that's the sort of thing you want." She notes that it can also leave your head spinning, giving examples of times she suggested an experiment Drucker thought had merit, but which needed additional support. He would make a few calls, and suddenly he had an international collaborator on board and a postdoc in that lab waiting to run the samples as soon as they were ready.

"It's like, whoa, we just had this idea 10 minutes ago, and now we're fully set up with a collaborator who's an expert in the field, and the limiting factor is me getting my samples," she says with a laugh. "That's the thing that makes working in his lab very exciting, but you have to be prepared to really pursue your questions."

It has also, she admits, set her up with some slightly unrealistic expectations now that she has her own lab. "Now I send an email to someone and wonder why I'm still waiting for a response 12 hours later," she says with a chuckle. Not everyone is as efficient as Drucker.

Dr. Elodie Varin, who came to Drucker's lab from France to complete her postdoctoral studies in 2013, agrees. After putting hours into preparing her cover letter and application, she assumed the chances that the world-renowned scientist would reply to an early-career trainee from a small lab in France were slim. "He actually responded within six minutes," she says, still incredulous, noting that he even apologized for the delay because he was in Japan. Within 30 minutes, she had secured a meeting with him during his upcoming trip to Paris.

"Thinking about it now, I believe the fact that I had been working on diabetes and incretins for several years showed I had a passion for this field," she says, noting that her technical skills also fit well with the needs of his team. "I think Dan wants the people who join his lab to have enough knowledge and expertise to be efficient and productive, but he also wants to make sure this will be a beneficial experience for them."

He was extremely invested in making sure she learned from her time working with him, she recalls, and even when she opted to leave to go into a career in scientific writing rather than start her own lab, Drucker was her biggest champion. His Twitter feed regularly lights up with supportive words and encouragement for scientists who opt to find ways to take their training beyond the traditional boundaries.

Like Mulvihill, Varin found Drucker's work ethic impressive. "He is always at least ten steps ahead of everyone," she says. "He works during the nights, the weekends, his holidays, the wedding day of his son. He is always there when you need him." In fact, she says, if you send a message to Drucker and he does not respond within ten minutes, you know he is on a plane without Wi-Fi—or on the golf course.

This responsiveness echoes my own experience. I did not even know Drucker *had* an assistant until many months into working on this book—and only then because I ran into her at an event. He set up all our meetings himself, and there was never a gatekeeper outside his office when I went to see him. He also answered my emails right away—even shocking me with detailed responses to questions I had sent only an hour after he received them, on a Saturday, from his cottage. No other researcher I have ever worked with is as responsive, yet Drucker's scientific output continues to be staggering.

He is dogged in his desire to continue to do excellent research, to help patients, to mentor young scientists, and to educate. For years, he has run his own lab website—an anomaly in the world of busy scientists, let alone legendary scientists of a certain age. Glucagon.com is an essential resource for those working in incretin biology, and his lab turns to it regularly.

"The page went down once while I was there, and it was paralysis for the Drucker Lab because that's where we get our information," notes Mulvihill, who is still in awe of the fact that her prestigious mentor is the one sitting at his desk fixing the home page because the site isn't working. "It's him. He's doing it. Not somebody else curating this research that he has outsourced to. No, It's him. And it is this massive resource, which is amazing when you're new to the field."

And while he may not delegate many of the tasks other senior scientists have long ago abdicated, there are still certain things that will cause him to drop everything—like his grandchildren. It's well-known in his lab that Drucker is always available unless his grandson needs a ride to music lessons, or there is a family event to attend. While as a parent Drucker may have spent the occasional weekend or evening dragging one of his sons along to his basement lab to check on experiments, he has become a bit more balanced with his time as he has aged.

"He's mellowed out a lot over the years. In just about every facet of his life, he's more relaxed," Drucker's son Aaron says. "He doesn't show up for work until around 10:30 a.m. in the summer because he's golfing for the first three hours of the day. And I think most people who know him as very hard working and not a super-relaxed guy would be surprised to hear that."

Not as shocking, what passes for relaxed in Drucker terms may not be quite what you'd expect. "Ever see someone literally running on a golf course with his golf bag on his shoulder and still playing faster than players using a golfcart?" asks Varin with a laugh. "Well, that's Dan."

* * * * *

Inspired by his accomplishments, more than one thousand health care professionals pack the hall for Drucker's presentation at Diabetes Canada's Professional Conference in November 2017. They are there to see him speak about his thirty-plus years of work in incretin biology, but it is his closing remarks—which he has become known for—that resonate the most. His impassioned reminder of the need for basic science funding is the thing that's on everyone's mind as they leave the room.

Now far enough into his career that he can speak freely, Drucker has a reputation as an advocate for basic and discovery-level science. He seems to relish his role as a champion for scientists who are doing the kind of work that helped him get to the stage where his own breakthroughs were possible. While he is happy to share these thoughts at a talk like this keynote, his platform is more often on Twitter these days.

Drucker has an outsized presence on social media. He tweets at a rate that makes you wonder just how many hours a day he has left to do the impressive amount of work he still produces. His typical posts talk about the latest research papers and events in the community. Sometimes he will quote pop culture in his microblogging with a very Drucker-ian aplomb, making me chuckle with references to everything from the Backstreet Boys to DeBarge in his descriptions of scientific studies. It's easy to imagine that somewhere, Sheldon Cooper from *The Big Bang Theory* is reading Drucker's latest missive and shouting, "Bazinga!"

He credits his daughter-in-law for his adoption of the medium. "If you asked me five years ago, 'Why don't you use Twitter to communicate your science and reach a broader audience?' I would have said, 'No, Twitter's ridiculous. It's just a social media channel that Beyoncé and Jay-Z use to tell us what they did on Saturday night. That's not a serious thing for scientists.'

"My daughter-in-law was probably 25 then, and she looked at me and said, 'You know, Dan, you're totally wrong. It's a really powerful communications medium. You can have a broad reach and really expand how you communicate your science. You should check it out.'"

Since this young woman worked at Google and was smart enough to marry his son, Drucker conceded that she probably understood social media better than he did. So, he decided to start an account, and he quickly realized she was right.

"At the end of the day, we come to work, we do our science, we have conventional ways that we handle our science, we go to meetings, we present abstracts, and we write papers or peer reviews that are published. And that is how we communicated science up until very recently," he says. "If you publish your paper in that journal, you'll probably have four or five hundred people seeing the paper when they do a literature search. Of those, one hundred or two hundred people might read it, and over time your work will be disseminated. But when I publish a paper on Twitter, by the time we get finished with Twitter stories, probably 25,000 or 50,000 people will have indirectly seen that paper. It's like a 100-fold difference in reach."

Beyond a place to raise awareness of his research, Twitter has also become a platform for Drucker to share his opinions with both his peers and the wider community. He has become a vocal advocate for issues that have a real impact on research—and more importantly—affect outcomes for patients.

Funding is always a struggle when it comes to research, and basic science is often the first to face cuts. This is frequently the source of his ire. The type of work on which Drucker has built his career is often also the most maligned. When critics look to cut "waste" in government spending, slow and methodical studies with uncertain outcomes and no promised glamourous breakthroughs are often the first on the chopping block.

The popular science podcast *Undiscovered* did an episode in their first season about American biologist Dr. Sheila Patek, who found herself defending work done in her lab about the mantis shrimp when a congressman listed it in his "wastebook" and likened it to using taxpayer dollars to pay for "shrimp fight club." For Patek, this small study was helping scientists better understand the unique properties of the mantis shrimp's tail, which acts as an extremely powerful hammer when used in defence. She was researching this in order to find practical human applications; having to explain and justify her work was a frustrating and time-consuming endeavour. However, it is an increasingly common occurrence for basic scientists.

Pharmaceutical companies interested in funding research want a quick return on investment. Telling them your project may or may not work out and that even if it does, it could be twenty years or more before it can be commercialized is not likely to get you an investor. But it's this sort of research that paves the way for those big discoveries—everything from vaccines to GPS and beyond began with someone somewhere doing basic science. For Drucker, this impatience on the part of funders is an ongoing source of frustration. He worries about how it will impact new investigators and future innovation.

"It's more difficult now than it has been in the last four decades to successfully transition from a period of training to an independent faculty position with a reasonably funded laboratory," he says. "Postdoctoral fellows spend longer periods of time training to try and make themselves more competitive. Many abandon their dreams to do science, faced with the reality of a low success rate and a harsh job market. We should formulate science policy based on real evidence of what works, and what the most successful countries do. We should not starve basic science based on fanciful ideas that politicians have about how to create and fund a strong knowledge economy."

It is not only the funding of research that has raised the ire of Drucker lately. He is equally frustrated at the lack of support he needs to get the drugs he worked so hard to develop into the hands of patients. GLP-1 agonists, you see, are not a pill that you swallow. Instead, they are a class of peptides (the building blocks that make up proteins in our bodies) dissolved in liquid that you inject under your skin. They may last for several days, and while they have been shown to be incredibly effective, they are also extremely expensive. In order to make the treatment available extensively, the organization that advises on drug reimbursements—in Canada, this is the Canadian Agency for Drugs and Technologies in Health (CADTH)—typically needs to approve that cost. And in the case of GLP-1 agonists, that has been taking a long time.

CADTH is a non-profit organization that assesses drugs and medical treatments, then provides information and recommendations to those making health care spending decisions about which treatments make the most sense for them to cover. In Canada, the provinces use these recommendations to decide which drugs and treatments make it onto their reimbursement plans—the ones accessible by seniors, those with low incomes, or those with specific conditions. These decisions also help determine what insurance companies are willing to cover.

Dr. Christopher McCabe, the chief executive officer of the Institute of Health Economics in Alberta, is an expert on how these sorts of decisions are made. I meet him at an event in Toronto, where he is speaking to a room full of stem cell scientists about the realities of whether or not their often extremely pricey therapies will ever be adopted by the Canadian system. In many cases, he tells them, they may simply be so expensive that they will never be widely available under the current health care plans.

It's hard for me not to think about Drucker as I listen to McCabe's talk, and afterwards, as we chat about how these decisions are made. I opted not to ask him specifically about GLP-1 agonists because, as I've learned in my research, decisions about funding a specific therapy are a moving target, and by the time this book reaches readers, GLP-1 agonists may be widely covered. As I type this, an oral version is already making inroads into the marketplace, and some versions are being tentatively covered in certain provinces.

Still, the premise of Drucker's argument—that the government and industry pump millions into funding research on new therapies that they then deem too expensive—is an ongoing source of frustration for scientists and not likely to change anytime soon, regardless of the status of one particular class of medications.

I wanted to better understand this rationale.

McCabe, who has served on the CADTH working group and helped author the fourth edition of their *Guidelines for the Economic Evaluation of Health Technologies* in 2017, understands the frustration. He encourages scientists to look at it from another viewpoint.

"I think of it this way: Efficacy is a *necessary* condition; value is a *sufficient* condition." In other words, does the good this new drug does outweigh the good of all the things that will have to be removed from the system in order to pay for it?

It's common to hear on the news about a drug or treatment that is desperately needed by a family with a sick child or a person who is dying—yet the cost of some of these miracle drugs can be astronomical. This all has to be weighed against the pot of money the province or system has available, McCabe explains, and whether providing this very expensive treatment for a small group justifies taking away other drugs or treatments from the larger group. It's a challenging call.

GLP-1 agonists are not the multimillion-dollar therapies we hear about on the news or something that your friend may be crowdfunding for on Facebook. They are simply good therapies that happen to be more expensive than the current, next-best options—and patients need to be on them long term, possibly for the rest of their lives, once they start treatment. GLP-1 agonists have been shown in studies to have better overall outcomes than sulfonylureas, the current approved therapy, but they are just more expensive.

For Drucker, who clearly understands that the pot of money to support new technologies is limited, restricting access and financial reimbursement to a well-established treatment with such positive long-term health benefits is shortsighted. Preventing access, he argues, will cause far more damage to the health of Canadians with diabetes, many of whom will have an increased risk of heart disease, stroke, or early death without this option.

The widespread good the treatment could provide, oddly enough, might be one of the biggest obstacles it faces in getting coverage. Type 2 diabetes is much more prevalent than a rare form of cancer. This means that, while the impact of a new medication on health care budgets may be relatively modest per person, when there are conceivably thousands of patients who will be taking this drug, the impact on budgets is potentially so large that it may not be sustainable.

McCabe explains that when a new treatment is being considered for coverage, the cost has to be in line with the least valuable thing on the coverage list. This means, basically, that those making the decision to cover GLP-1 agonists, must then remove other items from the list in order to make room for this new medication. A very expensive treatment that is used by a large number of people could potentially eat up funds that would otherwise go towards multiple other treatments.

The positive long-term outcomes of using GLP-1s are something that clinical trial after clinical trial has shown—these drugs help people with type 2 diabetes live longer, healthier lives, with fewer complications. I ask McCabe about how this knowledge factors into the budget process, as from my own simple math, it seems to make sense to invest in something that will have such large-scale benefits to health care costs in the long term.

He agrees in theory but notes that it all depends on how long down the road these impacts will be felt. With diabetes treatments that often don't show a return on investment until decades later, this can work against them.

"As human beings and societies, we don't value things that happen in the future as highly as we value things now. In economic evaluation, in all economics actually, we apply a weight that reflects the difference we attach to things, both positive and negative things, that happen in the future. So, if you prevent things that are forty, fifty years in the future, they get relatively small weight in the assessment."

He likens it to being asked if you would like $1,000 today or a promise of $1,000 in a year. Most of us would take the $1,000 now because we could invest it. And the future is uncertain. What if in a year from now, the person offering the $1,000 is unable to give it to you?

"There's good, rational reasons why benefits and costs that happen in the future do not get the same weight as things that are immediate," he says.

He also notes that often a drug will be brought in as a second-line for diabetes and is meant to be used after the very inexpensive and effective first-line therapy of metformin has proven to be inadequate for a patient's needs. But frequently, the new drug ends up being used far more widely than it was meant to be.

Physicians, eager to give their patients a therapy they consider superior, will often choose to start them on the much more costly treatment right away. This magnifies the impact on provincial budgets. While the doctor may simply be thinking about the best thing available for the patient in front of them, they often don't look at it through the lens of the long-term impact on the health care system and, hence other individuals' health.

Still, McCabe does offer hope. He notes that as other countries choose to start covering a treatment—something that continues to happen with many new diabetes therapies—there is much less risk in taking the chance on them. And as a therapy develops over time and gets closer to going off patent, the costs can become more sustainable. Ten years at full price without a generic option may be too much for the system to bear, but five or seven years considerably cuts down costs. Additionally, over time, the cost to manufacture a new treatment can become less expensive as the process becomes more streamlined and new technologies are developed to increase efficiency.

In the end, there are many things to consider about drug availabilities, and while CADTH plays an enormous role through informing governments about their options, McCabe notes that in the end, the provinces will make their own decisions. There are many drugs that have been approved by the organization or others tasked with this job, which still remain on a province's waiting list. Yet, ironically, others that the organization has suggested not be covered have ended up making the cut.

For Drucker, it's important to continue to pursue change. Not because he's unaware of why the decisions are being made, but because it all comes down to the reason he's devoted his life to research—to have a positive impact on the lives of people with diabetes. In his early years, he thought the goal was simply to figure out the science needed to develop the treatment, but now he knows he also has to invest time in ensuring it gets into the hands of those who can benefit from it.

"The whole GLP-1 story has made me very aware of how this works," he says. "What's the point of our government encouraging innovation, with science and bench-to-bedside translation, if when you finally have drugs that make a huge difference, another part of the system denies access? So, you have more heart attacks, more strokes, and more death? To me, that's a travesty."

And Drucker is, if nothing else, persistent in the face of adversity. It's a trait he comes by naturally. His parents are Holocaust survivors. His mother was born in Poland, and his father was raised in what was then Czechoslovakia. His mother was in prison or in hiding throughout the war, and most of her family were killed during this dark period in history. She arrived in Palestine as a refugee when the war ended. It was there she met Drucker's father, who had become part of a Czech brigade serving in the British army. Because he spoke multiple languages, Drucker Sr., whose father had been sent to Auschwitz and who had also lost much of his family during the war, had been asked to meet the refugee boats as they arrived. The couple met, fell in love, and then moved from Israel to Canada in 1953.

This history imbues Drucker's life and the determination which infuses his work. In many ways, I would argue it has also shaped his sense of social justice. Drucker was an early advocate for the ending of "manels"—conference panels made up almost entirely of men who were typically white—which were the norm for decades in science. He has also made a habit of hiring and mentoring some of the top female scientists in the world. Drucker sensed early on that women struggled to get placements in top labs, despite their talent, and that made it harder for them to get prestigious jobs after their postdoctoral studies. He has worked hard to change that.

This insistence on structural change is evident at his own events. At the annual Lunenfeld-Tanenbaum Research Institute's International Diabetes and Metabolism Symposium, which Drucker cochairs, he insists on having an equal number—if not more—female scientists present their research. On Twitter, he calls out those people who don't put in the same amount of effort. As he sees it, if you aren't having top female scientists present these days, you are not having the top *scientists* present.

Drucker is proud of the legacy he has created, noting the number of successful researchers who have come out of his lab. While he refuses to play favourites in terms of which, if any of them might succeed him, he is happy to laud all of their successes—and to fight for the resources they'll need to build on his accomplishments.

He simply hopes that those who make the decisions about who and what to fund look to the past and realize how important the initial work is to the end results. Advances like the ones he has made, or for that matter, the discovery of insulin, would not have been possible without support for fundamental science. Continued access to financial resources will be critical for younger scientists to make their own breakthroughs.

Many countries, he explains, fund basic science at much higher levels, relative to their GDP. He is deeply concerned that Canada will cease to be internationally competitive, despite having some of the best researchers in the world, if it does not reconsider the merits of funding basic science.

"The vast majority of breakthroughs in science, whether it is in physics, mathematics, engineering, biology, or chemistry, comes from unanticipated discoveries, often made by one or two individuals who stumble upon a key new concept due to their curiosity, imagination, and dogged pursuit of an interesting question," he says. "Simply review the list and history of Nobel Prize winners for evidence in support of how major discoveries were made."

Whether Canada's next Nobel will be found in the field of diabetes may just hinge on whether those who control the purse strings of science heed his warning.

An Unexpected Path to Excellence

Dr. Gary Lewis and his wife decided to come to Canada while watching the opening ceremonies of the 1988 Calgary Olympic Games. "They did this rodeo thing, and I thought, 'That looks like a nice place, maybe we'll go check it out,'" he recalls. Eighteen months later, he was applying for a job at the University of Toronto.

Like many of the defining moments in Lewis' career, it was something of a happy accident. "I'm a bit like Forest Gump; things just happen to me," he says, laughing, but there is a grain of truth in the analogy.

Born and raised in South Africa, Lewis had done his medical training there, but he knew that the country during Apartheid was not where he wanted to be. He applied for and received a residency position in Chicago, where he did three years of internal medicine.

His training in South Africa had been exceptional, but it was entirely clinical. Lewis loved being a physician, in particular, the interpersonal relationships the quick-witted doctor was able to build with a wide range of people. Yet, he felt the pull to do more. While he had no training or background in research, the idea of working in science intrigued him. "I just wanted to try it, check it out, see what it was about," he says. This is how he landed his first research position—reviewing charts for a staff hematologist—which he hated. The role was all wrong. He found the work boring and unstimulating, not allowing him to explore the deep curiosity and love of learning that fuels him.

Instead, he decided to focus on his clinical training and leave research to others. Then he applied for a fellowship position in the endocrinology department at the University of Chicago, and during the interview, they asked him why he wanted to pursue diabetes research. He had no idea. Lewis had not even realized the position involved research, and other than his disastrous time in a hematology lab, he had no experience in the area at all.

In the interview with the legendary Dr. Arthur Rubenstein, who was then the Chair of Medicine, Lewis remembers being completely thrown by the question. "I looked at him sort of quizzically and said, "Well, I'm not really committed specifically to diabetes research," he says now, laughing at the blunder. Rubenstein just looked at him and said, "Well, it sounds to me like you're not really committed to anything.'"

At that moment, Lewis remembers feeling like he was going to pass out, suddenly understanding that he was looking at an incredible career opportunity—and he was about to blow it. "My entire life came flashing in front of my eyes, and I realized with extreme clarity what I was applying for and what I should have said, and so I had to backtrack from that." He managed to pull himself together and said the things he should have said from the beginning, but the hiring committee wasn't interested in this clinician, who not only had almost no research experience, but who also had exactly *zero* diabetes research under his belt.

"They didn't really want me, but I was very persistent," he recalls. At the time, Lewis was doing very well in his residency, and he had all of his supervisors from the hospital call to recommend him. The hiring committee may not have wanted Lewis, but he had decided this was the role he was meant to have, and he was not going to give up easily. Eventually, he wore them down, landing the job and a role with one of the leading diabetes researchers of his time, Dr. Ken Polonsky.

Polonsky, realizing how green Lewis was in research, promptly sent the new hire to the library, where he spent three months figuring out a project. That time allowed Lewis to really refine the work he wanted to do and get his feet under him as he began three years in one of the world's top diabetes labs. "It was literally by just pure chance and totally not planned, and I started to do this very high-quality research," he says. "And of course, my experiments didn't work from the beginning, so I really learned the hard way."

Unlike his first research experience, though, Lewis found he loved this work. And after three years in Polonsky's lab, he was starting to make real progress. Unfortunately, the visa Lewis was studying under was not eligible for renewal, and he had to find a new position outside the U.S. or return to South Africa. Not interested in returning under Apartheid, and knowing if he did, he would have to go into mandatory military service, Lewis and his wife were weighing their options when they started watching the Calgary Olympics.

Like his previous experience in Chicago, Lewis was definitely not what the University of Toronto was looking for when he applied for a clinician-scientist position with the school. "I was by no means ready for a faculty position," Lewis admits. "I had only done three years of research."

Dr. Daniel Drucker, who was then a part of the hiring committee, had only agreed to interview the young scientist based on Polansky's recommendation. Lewis had little experience and no publications. Published research is how a scientist shows the value of their work, and as Drucker recalls, Lewis had only a few papers under review by journals when they met. Those publications Drucker thinks of as promissory notes. "They're what I call vapour papers," he says, likening it to when the software industry promises that version 2.0 will be out soon and offer so much more than the current version. "Sometimes, it would come out and be just like advertised, and other times, it would never come out."

Drucker recommended Lewis to the department head for a position based on his potential, however, and the strength of Polonsky's word—and hoped for the best. "You get lucky sometimes," he says of the decision. "Gary worked out really well, but not everyone's a Gary."

To say that Lewis worked out would be an understatement. The papers not only materialized and proved his academic mettle, but his research, which focuses on lipid metabolism, has become world leading. Several years after settling at the University of Toronto, he was tapped to become the head of the endocrinology division at the University Health Network. Later, he was appointed director of the University of Toronto's Division of Endocrinology, followed by an appointment to the role as the director of the Banting & Best Diabetes Centre, leading a group of some of Canada's best diabetes researchers. From there, he and Dr. Catharine Whiteside applied for and received funding to start Diabetes Action Canada, a patient-focused program that places those with diabetes at the heart of each and every research program.

Lewis describes the project as "the joy of my life." While the type of research he does—basic science in physiological models—doesn't lend itself easily to having a lot of patient-oriented research opportunities, he has discovered that the people who *live* with diabetes are an essential element of the research process—especially when moving a potential treatment out of the lab and into patients.

"I was very skeptical about patient engagement," he admits, "but we've learned. We have examples about how asking patients and engaging them deeply has changed the whole direction of a project. We have examples where we were going to do it one way, we were going to create a database this way, but patients said 'No, you're not, it's our data, and you're not going to do that.'"

There is little purpose in investing in research that does not meet the needs of those whose lives it seeks to improve, so this little project Lewis chose to invest his time in is now a huge part of his life's work.

Like everything in his career, Lewis sees this program as a part of the string of happy accidents that have led him to extraordinary things.

For the outside observer, it seems to be less accidental and more an example of how a smart, creative person can find their way to doing interesting and important things, even if they make mistakes or wander down the wrong path a few times on their way to figuring it all out. To those beginning their careers, Lewis' experience illustrates that you don't necessarily need to know where you will end up when you're starting out.

Lewis describes himself as lucky, having had a career where he's been able to work with so many talented and interesting people. He's inspired daily by not only the patients who inform research projects but also by the young scientists he's training and the many administrators and associates who make the programs he runs possible.

As he looks back, he's not quite sure why he chose medicine or science, but he knows that through a combination of luck, talent, privilege, and skill, he has made the most of it.

"They opened the door a crack, I pushed the door open, and they didn't have any choice. They couldn't get rid of me," he says, laughing. "I was very curious, I have a very high level of enthusiasm, and I just luckily enjoyed everything I did. Maybe if I'd been a welder, I would have loved welding, but whatever I did, I'd find the interesting aspects of it. I landed here, and the rest is history."

CHAPTER TWO

Do Research with Us, Not on Us

Dr. Christine Doucette is presenting to a room filled with trainees and investigators in Vancouver when she posts a slide that resonates with me in a way that rarely happens in a basic science presentation about the physiology of our cells.

She's talking about her work studying the beta cells of Indigenous communities in Northern Manitoba, where an unprecedented number of young people and children have been diagnosed with type 2 diabetes. The image shows the flat Prairie landscape of Manitoba, and she notes that less than 100 years ago, the people living on this land would have been eating a much different diet than they are now, post-colonization. Less than 100 years ago—not even two full lifetimes—everything was completely different for the people who lived and worked on this land. Looking at the image and thinking about just how short a time span 100 years is in evolutionary terms, it's easy to see why a population's genetic makeup may not have been able to keep up with the changes being forced upon them.

I've been talking to clinicians and scientists about the situation in Northern Manitoba for about as long as I've worked in the diabetes field. It's one of the most startling stories to come out of Canada— so much so that it was chronicled in the 2017 book *Diagnosing the Legacy: The Discovery, Research, and Treatment of Type 2 Diabetes in Indigenous Youth* by author Larry Krotz.

It was in Manitoba, in the mid-1980s, that Dr. Heather Dean and the pediatric diabetes team at the Children's Hospital of Winnipeg started to see a surprising phenomenon. Children from the province's remote Indigenous communities were being referred to her clinic with the symptoms of diabetes—but not type 1 diabetes, which was then considered the only form possible to develop in children.

Dean, who has since retired but remains a much-respected presence in the diabetes research community, was perplexed. She had opened the doors of the Diabetes Education Resource for Children & Adolescents clinic in 1985, and most of the province's 400 to 500 children with type 1 diabetes had transitioned there from the Children's Hospital. A few were from Northern communities, but these young people seemed different.

In type 1 diabetes, there is weight loss, fatigue, intense thirst, and frequent urination. A1C (average blood sugar) levels are high and can only be managed through insulin injections. These children from the North tended to carry much more weight, and it seemed counter-intuitive to treat them with insulin. Many refused to take it, anyway—and they displayed none of the typical symptoms. "The first one scared me because I had no idea," Dean admits, shocked to see a young girl of just fifteen with a blood sugar of 25 when a normal level should be between four and seven.

Then another young person came into the clinic with similar symptoms, and another, and another. After almost a dozen presented at her clinic within just a few years, Dean decided she needed to go up North and speak with the community. She wanted to know more about what was going on and also to seek their guidance. Community is key in Indigenous populations, and she knew that this problem could not be managed without a better understanding of what was happening. They needed to work together to find a solution.

"None of the methods we use for adults can be used in these kids," she says, speaking of the medications and lifestyle modification suggestions that are most often advised when people are diagnosed with type 2 diabetes. For children in remote Manitoba communities, the situation was much more complex.

Dean didn't know during that initial visit that working with these young people and these communities would become her life's work.

She had a moment similar to the one I experienced during Christine Doucette's presentation many years earlier, but hers was much more profound. In the 1930s, Dean's father had spent several years working for the Hudson's Bay Company as a fur trader in Northern communities. When she found out about this as an adult—already working in Indigenous child health with many of these same communities—she invited him to join her on a trip she was taking to Big Trout Lake in Northern Ontario. Her father had spent time there while working in the fur trade, and Dean thought it would be interesting to see the community through his eyes.

"We were talking about his time in Big Trout Lake and how at that time there were only two buildings. One was the Hudson's Bay Company, and one was the church," she recalls. The rest of the community was still in tents. "To see Big Trout with houses, a nursing station, a store, and a school was quite a surprise. He knew that there had been development, clearly, but it was so different than in 1937 when he was up there."

Her father showed her where he would hunt rabbits and where he had worked. Looking around at the community in 2002 and thinking about her father's view from 1937 was a stark reminder of how quickly change had come to this part of the world. "It hit me like a rock that it's so recent, and it's not surprising that diabetes wasn't seen then. Everyone was out on the land. I knew that from my history books, but it wasn't real," she says.

The turnabout from traditional culture came quickly—and without much thought to the impact on the Indigenous communities. This is something Dean and those who have joined in her work know all too well. While there is no single answer to why Indigenous children and youth began to develop type 2 diabetes, there is an understanding that the confluence of elements that came with colonization all play a role.

The loss of culture, residential school trauma, housing insecurity, limited access to healthy food, and the change from a traditional to Western diet have severely altered a community where the most devastating effects of diabetes are being seen in younger and younger members of the population.

Dean spent years working together with the communities hardest hit by type 2 diabetes diagnoses in children. She joined leading researchers Dr. Stewart Harris and Dr. Bernard Zinman—who had been studying the epidemic of type 2 diabetes in Indigenous communities in Sandy Lake, Ontario—to share and exchange information. And then she began to publish papers on what she discovered. Dean knew it was critical to spread the word about what she was seeing— not only to gain additional insights from other scientists, but also to establish that something rare was happening in these communities, and if nothing was done, the consequences for future generations of Indigenous youth could be dire.

That she was able to get anything about this topic published in a scientific journal at the time is a testament to her tenacity and skill. "My mentor and my research training were not in diabetes," she explains.

This made her an unlikely candidate to publish on a new phenomenon in the field. In fact, she faced a wall of disbelief when she and her team started to raise the alarm about what they were seeing in these northern communities, as type 2 diabetes had never previously been observed in children and young adults. Others in the diabetes field assumed she was just missing the signs of what had to be type 1 diabetes.

But as her team amassed more and more evidence, the research community slowly started to come around to the idea. "I came in through the back door. Basically, everything I did was just observational in the beginning," says Dean, who began her research in the area by simply reporting what she was seeing in her clinic. What she was discovering was new, however, which made it easier to publish, but she still faced pushback.

"The very first paper I published was in the *Canadian Medical Association Journal* in 1992. I had a hard time getting that published because the reviewers said, 'How do you know it's not early type 1 diabetes?'"

Her experience of treating and interacting with these children was not enough evidence in and of itself, and so she was asked to resubmit her work once she had more quantifiable evidence, such as tests showing that these children did not have the antibodies associated with type 1 diabetes. This was a difficult task at the time due to the technological limitations of that type of testing, but one she was able to achieve with the support of a colleague from Boston.

Dean still faced resistance, though, as the scientific community remained hesitant to accept a phenomenon that seemed only to exist in these remote, isolated communities. She continued to plug away regardless, publishing her findings, presenting at conferences, and working intently with the children and families who were coming to her clinic in increasingly large numbers.

In the mid-1990s, Dean was invited to the Centers for Disease Control and Prevention (CDC) in Atlanta, where she and a group of other researchers from around the world were asked to work with the organization's epidemiologists to try and determine how to differentiate type 1 diabetes and type 2 diabetes in children.

At the time, her findings were still not accepted by the American Diabetes Association, which publishes the American guidelines for diabetes treatment and care, so the CDC invitation was a welcome one. In Atlanta, Dean worked with other clinicians and scientists who were seeing a similar phenomenon in marginalized communities—Indigenous, African American, Asian, Latino, and others. They observed similar characteristics like family history, obesity, and being part of Indigenous or minority populations as factors that were associated with youth-onset type 2 diabetes. The work, however, still had a long way to go.

"We had this series of indicators, that if you had them, you were most likely going to have type 2 diabetes," Dean recalls of the process. "That was before we had a good assay for antibodies, which is now what we use to confirm a type 1 diabetes diagnosis, but in the early days, it was hard. My research was purely out of an innate curiosity and a drive to help because I didn't know how to help these kids and these communities. Nor did I know what to *tell* the communities."

Dean could see that the Elders and families understood what was happening, and she was driven to continue her work alongside them to find solutions.

Her research in this area could in and of itself fill a book—see the aforementioned *Diagnosing the Legacy: The Discovery, Research, and Treatment of Type 2 Diabetes in Indigenous Youth*, which I highly recommend—but while understanding and acceptance of this diagnosis has changed since those first young people stepped into her clinic, there is still much to figure out for those who are now following in Dean's footsteps.

This next generation of scientists is aptly named the "DREAM network," which stands for Diabetes Research Envisioned and Accomplished in Manitoba. The group is made up of a host of clinicians and scientists working together with the province's Indigenous communities to achieve better treatments and to increase prevention, where possible.

Many of those initial children who were seen by Dean in the 1990s have since gone on to have their own children, and now a third generation of diabetes is starting to emerge. These children, born of mothers and grandmothers who were diagnosed with the disease in youth, are in many cases developing diabetes themselves at even earlier ages. Dean and her colleagues, including Dr. Elizabeth Sellers, Dr. Brandy Wicklow, and Dr. Allison Dart, have been able to follow these families and map the progress of diabetes as it travels from generation to generation. Following Dean's retirement, Wicklow has stepped up to lead the research arm of this project, the Next Generation Birth Cohort.

Wicklow is, in many ways, Dean's polar opposite. Dean has retired to farm life, fitting in perfectly with her jeans, flannel shirt, and greying hair cut in a sensible bob. Wicklow, on the other hand, wears sleek black heels and pencil skirts when she presents her research. Where Dean seems practical and patient, Wicklow laughs loudly and easily, exuding a warmth that is hard to resist. When she wraps me in a hug at the end of our first meeting, after trading her heels for more practical flats to walk to her hotel, it feels both genuine and endearing.

Both women share a whip-smart intelligence and a desire to effect change, as well as the tenacity to make it happen. There is a reason they have been embraced so warmly by the Indigenous community they work alongside. They are not there to tell anyone what to do, but instead to listen, learn, and provide whatever tools they can offer in this fight. This has been at the heart of the program's success and has provided Wicklow with the enviable gift of a cohort—a group of people who she has been able to study over the course of their lifespan. It's allowed her to look through a window into three generations of type 2 diabetes in this population and has given her the ability to study what's happening in these communities with an unparalleled level of granularity.

Her work would not be possible if those in the community did not welcome her. The families first treated by Dean are now seen by Wicklow. She flies into the communities to meet them four times a year, and the youth travel to her twice a year. When someone from her cohort becomes pregnant, they know to keep her updated, and they recognize that she needs certain things to continue to study and learn. The community wants to be a part of understanding the impact on their lives and those of their children.

Many of the original women who Dean worked with or who were treated by her have now passed on, often from diabetes complications, but their children and grandchildren continue to support the programs. "They are so good—having known that their mothers were involved with us," says Dean. "The challenge is actually reminding them in the excitement of having a baby that we need to have all of this stuff done, too, like the cord blood for Brandy. But if Brandy calls, they know the history of their mother and their grandmother, and it's a lovely long story of partnership and friendship."

For Wicklow, working with these families and being so deeply embedded in their lives fuels her love for the work. "I think that's where the passion comes from—seeing families and getting to meet families and know them as a unit. As a family structure and as a community structure. It's remarkable how generous they are with their time. How generous they are in terms of letting us know what it's like to live with diabetes. I spend a lot of time engaging with them about what's meaningful research and what are the relevant questions. And then, how do we interpret the results we're getting, and how can we best share those results with the families and community members? We have a very dedicated group of kids and parents who have worked with me now for ten years to do just that. I think it makes the work more important, but I also think it makes it more rewarding for me because it feels like a partnership. We're working through this problem together. It's phenomenal. I wouldn't want to do research any other way."

That feeling also translates over to the basic science side of things. While Wicklow and Dean are clinicians who do research, they also understand the need for basic scientists to help explain the findings they are bringing forward. And in the DREAM structure, basic scientists are not simply sitting in their labs looking at cells in a dish.

* * * * *

I'm having breakfast with Dr. Christine Doucette the morning before she gives her keynote address to a crowded room at the University of British Columbia. We're talking about the interesting things coming out of nutritional science—the way scientists are starting to use physiology to determine who would benefit from eating what. We both struggle with this because of a deep understanding of the barriers that make eating based on what science says is best nearly impossible.

Doucette grew up in Scarborough, Ontario, a suburb of Toronto, where I was also born and raised. With her bouncy blonde curls and easy laugh, she reminds me of many of those I grew up with. Scarborough in the 1980s and '90s was a mix of working-class families, new Canadians, and those who veered toward a slightly upper-middle class. There is a street-smart wisdom and a practical veneer that many of us seem to have adopted, regardless of where we ended up in life, and it's easy to see that in Doucette.

In a few minutes, she will give a talk about physiology and her own findings on changes to the body based on the transition from a traditional to a Western diet. But she is acutely aware that there are more pressing needs with most of the patients her team sees than understanding what they should and should not eat.

She tells me the story of a young teenage girl she met at an event for Indigenous youth. The teen came to the clinic in flip-flops. In winter. In Manitoba. Just the thought of this is enough to leave me shivering, but for this girl, who may not have had other shoes, this might not have been just a fashion choice. Doucette, an avid runner, went to her office and brought back her running shoes, which were close enough to a fit to work.

There is no way you can look at a young person who may not have access to proper footwear, and explain what foods they should be eating or the type of exercise they need to be doing to stave off type 2 diabetes. No matter what Doucette sees through her microscope, that teenage girl will always be in the back of her mind, reminding her that it's about more than just the basic science.

Doucette is another researcher building on the foundation laid by Dean. When work began in Indigenous communities, blood samples were taken, and there was the recognition that a certain marker— a variant in the HNF1-alpha gene—seemed to be present in many of those who developed diabetes. At the time, the technology hadn't evolved enough to understand what this might mean. Now, scientists like Doucette can use the latest gene-editing technologies to reverse engineer this gene variant in cells and in mice in order to try and determine how it might create a predisposition to developing type 2 diabetes, and importantly, how it interacts with diet to increase susceptibility and early onset of diabetes in these Indigenous communities.

In her lab, Doucette is looking at different aspects of type 2 diabetes to figure out why pancreatic beta cells stop producing enough insulin. She is observing circadian rhythms and insulin secretion, as well as genetic variants and diet, and how these can all contribute to the onset of type 2 diabetes in youth. Understanding this complicated process and basic biology provides the foundation for the clinical practice. Her integration into the research program in Manitoba is critical to its success.

"One of the reasons I was very excited about moving to Manitoba to begin my research there was because of people like Brandy Wicklow and Heather Dean, who have spent their careers doing the clinical work and describing the situation of what these kids actually look like in the clinic," Doucette says. "Because of what they've been able to convey to us, we can basically reverse engineer what they're seeing [in patients] in our animal models."

These animal models play an important role in helping a researcher study how diabetes develops and progresses. This process has led to a strong collaboration between Doucette and Wicklow who—despite the very different types of work they do—are able to develop new and better strategies by working together. Wicklow brings what she's learning through her clinics to Doucette, who in turn, can explain the molecular processes she's finding. It's the ultimate bench-to-bedside translational work that often leads to great scientific breakthroughs.

"I think collaboration is fundamental now for any kind of research," says Wicklow. "I can't do the mechanistic studies. I'm a clinician, and so in terms of a cure or pharmaceutical treatment, those things are made in labs, at benches." Those discoveries come through conversation and consultation with those who are seeing the issues in the clinic. It is a cycle that, when honed, can reap great results.

Some of those who are now a fundamental part of the DREAM team did not envision that this was where they would end up. Dr. Jon McGavock planned to be a gym teacher, but when he started his kinesiology studies and saw how exercise could impact health outcomes, his focus shifted. His exuberance for his work is offset by the air of hipster cool that surrounds him, and he has become a leading voice on exercise and diabetes—both for type 1 and type 2. He has also become ingrained in the Indigenous communities that he works with, and it's easy to see why the youth would gravitate toward him.

McGavock grew up in Winnipeg's economically disadvantaged North End, and he understands the world-weariness of many that come from there. Despite not being Indigenous himself, he has listened to those in the community to try and understand how to make his own work relate to those who might have bigger concerns than how much time they spend being physically active in a week.

"By the time I came to the scene, type 2 diabetes in youth was on the radar, but people weren't really sure what was happening. At our centre, when I first started, I would say 95 percent of the children who were coming to the Children's Hospital to be treated for type 2 diabetes were Indigenous. A lot of them were in Northern communities, and that comes with all of the things that those communities are experiencing: the legacy of colonialism, institutional racism, the atrocities of the past, and the current challenges they face with regards to food security and poverty, and those sorts of things," he says. "It opened up an entire new area of research, and for me personally, an entire new viewpoint on Canada and the history of Canada."

I have often said that I should never spend time around McGavock while in possession of my credit card, because his sincere passion for the work he does makes you want to hand over all your money to support the change he wants to see in the world. Whether he is working to improve the biking trails in Manitoba for the betterment of the entire community or spending time with Indigenous youth to more fully understand how to create interventions that support their needs, he has the sort of optimism with an edge of reality that is hard to ignore.

"I think we always tend to lean towards the easy answer. We want a simple solution," he says of the type 2 diabetes increase being seen in Manitoba. There are many people who would love to blame it all on what kids are eating. "What we really need are the stories of youth. We need their voices to talk to us about their situation. And I'll give you a great example of how that impacts their health and how we deliver health care to these children.

"A paper we published in *The Lancet* showed that 40 to 60 percent of youth living with diabetes live in poverty, which means there may be days in the month when there might not be enough food in the household. We know that food insecurity is common in people with type 1 and with type 2, but if you go see your health care provider and they show you a food portion plate and say, 'Oh, you should have mostly fruit and vegetables, then some carbohydrate, then some meat,' but you haven't had food in your house for two days, how do you think that message is going to be received by that child? And do you think that adopting healthy behaviours that are out of their reach is going to be something that's possible? Collectively, that also leads to a bit of stigma. By just focusing on diet, you're sending the message that we think you're not eating healthy. If the youth themselves are thinking about the amount of money in the house, the amount of food in the house, other trauma that they're facing, and we don't acknowledge that or bring that to the table; we'll never get to the point where we can start to improve the health of these children."

Wicklow sees all of these issues in her work. Diabetes in Indigenous children and youth runs far deeper than genetics. "I think the mistake would be to say that First Nations people are at higher risk of developing diabetes because they are First Nations. We are 99.9 percent the same in terms of the human genome project," she says. "There are some good studies to say that in places where culture and language have been preserved, diabetes rates are actually lower in Indigenous populations.

"There are also other components of health in terms of belonging and knowing culture or practicing culture—whatever that looks like for your family—family function, community function, and support that play a role in diabetes risk and how well you live with diabetes if you have it. So, should you develop diabetes, you need all of those things around you to sort of wrap around you to help you get through that chronic illness and live with it as well as you can. Then, when you have your own children, you're in a healthy state, which helps you pass less of that risk on. So that's sort of the bigger, intergenerational picture, but there are important socioecological and historical data to incorporate into all studies that look at why one population is at a higher risk than another."

This way of looking at the issues facing youth with type 2 diabetes has permeated even more of the work being done by the DREAM team. Many of the youth being treated for diabetes also struggle with kidney disease. This means multiple appointments and trips to Winnipeg for young people who are already dealing with many challenges. The team, led by Wicklow and Dr. Allison Dart, decided instead to create a program that combined both the diabetes and kidney treatments into one clinic visit, paired with a sharing circle and an art component. The goal of the program, Wicklow explains, is to reduce power differentials and improve comfort and safety for patients.

There are eight kids per clinic who are seen every three months—a total of twenty-four youth altogether—and they arrive early in the morning to participate in a sharing circle with an Elder, who speaks Cree. This shared language helps families to contribute their thoughts and feelings comfortably. Wicklow and Dart participate in the circle as well, and in the art or other projects that take place during that first hour. After that, the kids move on to the diabetes and kidney treatments, but it allows for a sense of community and starts the day out in a way that supports more than just their physical well-being.

"That's a huge step and will expand in the future as more and more people recognize the value of that hour to the therapeutic side of things," says Dean. "Because for the next two hours, they're in clinic, looking at their kidney function and their diabetes, which is the last thing those kids want to do, so I think that first hour is beautiful."

The next step may be an expansion of that program, or it may go in different directions, depending on the community's needs. One thing that is certain is that more of the voices on the health care side will be Indigenous. This is something integral to the process and which has been a priority since the earliest days of the program when Dean hired Bertha Flett. It was Flett who helped create connections and understanding between the health care workers and the community, which was pivotal for establishing trust and support. Now, more and more youth from Indigenous communities are becoming part of the health care teams and determining how the process should develop.

The mantra of "nothing about us without us" infiltrates all areas of the work being done by DREAM, and there is a sense of pride and acknowledgment as more and more Indigenous health care workers are joining their ranks. One of the most promising voices is Taylor Morriseau, who joined the team as a PhD student in the labs of Christine Doucette and Vern Dolinsky.

Morriseau is Cree and belongs to the Peguis First Nation. Growing up in Manitoba, she felt a strong urge to find ways to support and nurture her community. A co-op placement led her to the research lab and an understanding of how to use science to help those with diabetes. When she decided to pursue graduate studies, hoping to have a career working in Indigenous health, she assumed that would mean leaving the province. Instead, a mentor pointed her towards DREAM. For Morriseau, who felt conflicted about leaving the community she wanted to help, it was the perfect fit.

The team is lucky to have her. The tiny, soft-spoken Morriseau has not even completed her PhD when I first meet her, and yet she has already made a significant contribution to the work being done in Manitoba. Doucette credits her with bringing a critical Indigenous lens to their work looking at the importance of a traditional diet.

Morriseau's work as a mentor for Indigenous youth has also earned her a wealth of accolades. When I interview her for this book, she has recently returned from a trip to Toronto, where she was named one of Canada's Most Powerful Women by the Women's Executive Network. She has also been named one of Manitoba's Top 30 Under 30 Sustainability Leaders by Corporate Knights, a CBC Manitoba Future 40 award winner, and is a Vanier scholar. For Morriseau, it's critical that Indigenous Peoples should play a part in the work being done to manage the diabetes epidemic in Manitoba.

In the lab, Doucette is one of the most accomplished scientists in Canada. Her work is well-funded, which allows her team to have access to the tools they need to do the best science possible. However, she cannot see things through the same lens that Morriseau has as an Indigenous person who comes from the community being studied. "I think it's been a really interesting relationship having a non-Indigenous and an Indigenous person come at the same problem together and bring unique perspectives," Morriseau says.

She also appreciates that the DREAM researchers understand and respect the complex reality that Indigenous communities face. Here, no one disputes that colonization, institutionalized racism, loss of culture, and many other factors play a role in the diabetes epidemic.

"It's sometimes so hard to convey to a basic science audience why they need to understand colonization from the 1600s and beyond. It doesn't click right away," she says. "But if everyone is already on the same page, and that's true for the DREAM network, conversations just pick up so quickly, and advance the research so much faster. For myself, it's fascinating because having everybody have that knowledge of history makes it a safer working environment in general."

Now a mentor and role model herself, Morriseau is helping a new generation of Indigenous youth make decisions about their future. While she has been buoyed by seeing those she has mentored pursue university degrees or study medicine, she explains that it's more complicated than just advocating for young people to move on to higher education. The barriers faced by Indigenous youth must be considered, as well as the reality that if every bright young mind leaves the community, it creates a brain drain that will impact the ability to do the work needed. "Sometimes we need people to stay in the community and help it prosper," she says.

Even the research she and Doucette are bringing forward about traditional diets cannot happen simply by telling people what they've discovered. "If I'm saying traditional foods in the lab are fantastic, there has to be youth and leaders who are engaged and willing to start up a hunting program or do a traditional food bank, all working together," Morriseau explains. "Having community-based research or community-based programs led by the youth in the community— that's what I hope for. At the end of the day, I hope youth can stay in the community, make investments in that community, and live healthy lives."

For Dean, watching closely as the next generation develops, having Indigenous scholars on board is simply the only way forward. She notes that one of her pediatric residents, who is Métis, recently moved into emergency medicine because it left her more time to do clinics in Northern Manitoba. Dean sees this same drive in researchers like Morriseau, who are drawn to the work by a keen sense of wanting to help their communities. "I think having more and more people who have a passion for Indigenous child health will help everybody," she says.

And when I ask Morriseau what she sees as the future of diabetes research in Canada, she is clear. "I think it requires intense, interdisciplinary collaboration," she says. "You can't answer a question like diabetes with just basic science. It's just impossible. You can't answer a multi-factorial problem with one single discipline. Having that array of different sciences, whether informational interviews with qualitative science or working with a mouse model like I do, however you approach the problem, do it together. But also, do it with a new generation of Indigenous scholars leading the way, especially when it comes to Indigenous diabetes in children. Have Indigenous scholars ask the right questions and lead that conversation, but also speak with really intelligent non-Indigenous counterparts. I think that will be the next wave."

CHAPTER THREE

It's Complicated

On February 13, 1967, Beth Mitchell got the diagnosis that would forever alter her life. She was eight years old and recovering from a mild case of the mumps when doctors discovered she had type 1 diabetes. Back then, it was called juvenile diabetes, as it was mainly diagnosed in children. There were no continuous glucose monitors or insulin pumps, no long-lasting insulin or even test strips. Mitchell had to use urine dip tests to check her sugar levels and glass syringes to inject insulin. She needed to match her mealtime insulin doses to "food exchanges," allowing her a specific number of carbohydrate, protein, and fat exchange "units" per meal and per day. Even now, more than fifty years later, she can automatically calculate in her head that fourteen grapes equal one carbohydrate food exchange.

When I meet Mitchell in the spring of 2018, I like her immediately. She is a firecracker of a woman, full of energy and eager to share her story about living with a condition which, had she developed it only a few decades before her diagnosis in the 1960s, might have been a death sentence. She is a retired schoolteacher now, having had a long career with the Toronto District School Board, and we have to arrange our meeting around her hectic schedule. She is a member of Toronto's Dragons Abreast dragon boating team and was an avid runner for decades. She looks nowhere near her fifty-nine years.

We are meeting to discuss her role in the Canadian Study of Longevity in Type 1 Diabetes project. The name is a mouthful, but its purpose is an important one. The researchers involved are trying to determine why some people who develop type 1 diabetes suffer more negative consequences from the disease—devastating complications like kidney failure, blindness, and amputations—while others, like Mitchell, seem to thrive, despite nearly a lifetime of type 1 diabetes. To be clear, no one who lives with type 1 diabetes has an easy road ahead. It involves constant management and is a 24-7 job, from which there are few breaks. But why do some people who have the disease seem to avoid the most insidious complications, while others don't?

Of course, how you manage your diabetes definitely factors in. Some people are simply able to do a better job of taking care of themselves, but in other cases, there seems to be no rhyme or reason when it comes to who will be hit with nerve damage, vision loss, or other serious complications.

To try to figure this out, researchers at Toronto's Lunenfeld-Tanenbaum Research Institute have undertaken what's called an observational cohort study. That's a somewhat complicated way of saying they're analyzing people who have had the disease for more than fifty years, running tests and having participants fill in detailed questionnaires about their medical history, how they manage their diabetes, and any obstacles they have experienced along the way. The purpose is to try and identify why some people with the disease develop complications. If researchers can answer this central question, they can then potentially develop treatments to ward off these additional burdens.

Leading this study is one of the world's foremost experts in diabetes complications—a researcher from Toronto whose mission it is to make the day-to-day life of people with diabetes easier to manage. He understands their struggles better than most, given his unique perspective.

Dr. Bruce Perkins is one of those people who is almost preternaturally gifted. Tall, handsome, and athletic, he's the sort of guy who, when he received a type 1 diabetes diagnosis at age eighteen, worried it would prevent him from keeping up with his peers and reaching his goals—then determined that it most certainly would not.

Instead, he scrapped his dream of studying veterinary science and working with wild animals in Africa and decided to attend medical school. He graduated from the University of Toronto with his medical degree, then went on to earn a Master's degree in public health from Harvard University. When he set out to study complications from diabetes, he quickly rose to the top in his field.

Perkins is the type of guy who leads the medical team when a group of people with type 1 diabetes climbs Mount Kilimanjaro and then Machu Picchu. He then co-authors a highly regarded paper about the effects of altitude on insulin resistance. He is also the sort of person who takes up golf as a kid and goes on to play competitively.

When he is asked to pick walk-on music for a plenary speech at a conference, he opts instead to perform a pitch-perfect version of Leonard Cohen's "Hallelujah" and accompanies himself on guitar before giving his hour-long talk. He is also the type of man who, when I suggest moving away from the impressive painting on his office wall during a video shoot because of copyright concerns, promises not to sue me. Because he painted it. Of course he did.

Bruce Perkins is ridiculously accomplished, but it's hard not to like him. He is the first to volunteer (and often over-volunteer) when called on to help the diabetes community. He says "Yes" when other researchers with half his prestige beg off because of other commitments, and he does it all with a smile on his face—and a self-deprecating sense of humour.

Much of what drives Perkins is his determination to understand and lessen the impact of diabetes complications. "Anyone with diabetes should be able to lead a life as creative, adventurous, challenging, and wonderful as in a parallel life without diabetes," he says. To do that, he firmly believes they need to avoid complications.

And while a great deal of work has been done in search of a cure and toward finding better treatments, when Perkins first started looking for information about complications, he discovered a huge gap. "I was shocked to learn as I got into this career that in many aspects of complications, we don't even understand basic things, like how to identify them," he says. "How can we tell that someone is developing early stages of eye, kidney, nerve, and cardiovascular damage? If we can identify these things earlier, there's more we can do to prevent them from getting worse, as opposed to only identifying things when it's too late. If we wait too long as a person with diabetes develops a complication, we then need miracles in terms of treatments, to try and reverse them from advanced stages."

The Canadian contribution has been significant when it comes to the work that has already been done on diabetes complications. The Diabetes Control and Complications Trial (DCCT) is an international study that has been running since 1982. Funded and run by the National Institutes for Health (NIH) in the United States, it poses the question as to whether the long-term complications of diabetes could be better managed through improved glucose control.

Dr. Bernard Zinman, a Toronto-based endocrinologist and researcher, was part of the original group of DCCT investigators funded in 1982 and has spent more than thirty years working on the project, including as chair of the Publication Committee and vice-chair of the Steering Committee. This study has been critical in proving that maintaining good glucose control could slow the progress of diabetes complications like kidney disease, vision loss, heart disease and nerve damage. It has also had huge implications on how type 1 diabetes is managed and treated today.

"I'm very fortunate because it's rare in a scientific career that you get to have an impact that changes how diabetes is treated. The DCCT study results dramatically established a new standard for how we manage type 1 diabetes," says Zinman. The study is one of the longest-running in NIH history, allowing the researchers to see the impact of improved glucose control over not just years but decades. "It also demonstrated what we called metabolic memory or a legacy effect," explains Zinman. This means that early glucose control is essential and has a long-lasting effect in reducing the development of future complications.

On some levels, this may seem somewhat disheartening, especially as experts know that young people with type 1 diabetes often go through a phase—in particular in their late teens and early twenties—when their blood sugar control wanes as they go through the typical rites of passage of adolescence. The DCCT, however, opened the door to a new generation of research and education around the importance of tight glycemic control and how to better manage these transitional stages of life.

Zinman's contributions to this research have been widely recognized, and he has gone on to work on other seminal trials, earning international acclaim and paving the way for researchers like Perkins to delve even deeper into understanding the outcomes of diabetes over the lifespan.

"When the DCCT was published, I was in medical school, and this study had the biggest impact on my understanding of complications," says Perkins. "I realized with one hundred percent certainty that my research would revolve around working to ensure people living with diabetes could avoid the fear of complications."

Unlike some scientists, Perkins is also a practicing endocrinologist, seeing patients as often as he can, given the competing needs of his lab and his roles as director of the Leadership Sinai Diabetes Centre and a professor of medicine at the University of Toronto. He says that working with patients gives him a different perspective on their needs, and his passion for his work is driven by those interactions.

"When I see someone who handles neuropathy, kidney disease, hypoglycemia, or their day-to-day blood sugars, and I see how they respond to hearing that their A1C [blood sugar level] is much higher than they thought it was, these are the things that drive me to do research that's a lot more practical and applied," he says. "There are other scientists out there in discovery research, where their goal is not actually meant to help patients today. It's meant to give them hope that tomorrow or in some years' time, there might be a cure. The kinds of skills I have are less so in that domain. I'm going to leave that to the brilliant researchers who are going to cure this disease. For me, I'm interested in things that, in the short term, could really help a generation of people with diabetes, and how they can manage it better day by day and prevent complications."

This is what has driven Perkins in the Longevity Study, as well as a host of other research projects all aimed at helping people *now*. It is a common refrain of those living with type 1 diabetes that they are constantly reading headlines or coming across news that a cure is imminent. They have heard countless times that some scientist somewhere has "cured diabetes in the lab," which is to say that they have cured diabetes in animal models—a far cry from curing it in humans. Yet for someone like Beth Mitchell, who has lived with diabetes for more than fifty years, or even Perkins himself, who has had the disease for more than thirty years now, a cure being discovered in their lifetime is not a given.

"Over the time in my life that I've had diabetes, I've heard of potential cures and gotten very excited about them," says Perkins. "Yet, the condition is not cured now." This, he explains, does not mean that the discovery-level science being done towards a cure isn't incredibly important—it is—but he believes we have to accept that this cure might not happen as quickly as we'd hope.

The extensive research on diabetes done in labs all over the world during the last few decades means that Mitchell and Perkins, and the other estimated 300,000 Canadians living with type 1 diabetes, now have access to insulin pumps, continuous glucose monitors, higher-quality insulins, and a host of other advances that make the day-to-day management easier. Through his research, Perkins would like to see even more forward movement—things that not only reduce the burden of living with diabetes but also lessen the fear of complications.

His first major foray into this was in the area of kidney disease. As with many complications, Perkins found that there were no good indicators that someone would develop kidney disease until the condition had progressed to a certain point. Through extensive study, he and his research collaborators were able to identify new causal factors and ways to identify subtle changes in renal function. It was a start. From there, he cast his eye on diabetic neuropathy—or nerve damage—which is responsible for one of the most dreaded diabetes complications—amputation.

Alongside Toronto's Dr. Vera Bril, Perkins was part of the team that developed the Toronto Clinical Scoring System for Diabetic Polyneuropathy, which helps to identify and diagnose neuropathy in patients earlier and with more accuracy. The system has been widely adopted by the research community internationally and has helped to considerably improve care in this area. Still, it wasn't enough for Perkins, who felt that finding out who was likely to develop neuropathy before it started was key to changing the lives of people living with diabetes. His enthusiasm for potential early identifiers, like corneal confocal microscopy—a very clinical way of saying the ability to diagnose diabetic nerve damage early by studying the cornea—can be infectious.

"The odd irony about nerve damage is that in a life with diabetes, probably everyone will get some degree of damage to their peripheral nerves," he explains. "Even though it's one of the most common complications of diabetes, it's also sort of forgotten, or not emphasized. I think in part it's because we haven't got good ways of identifying and measuring it."

And neuropathy isn't a benign condition. Some people who develop it will find the numbness in their feet distracting or painful, and it often interferes with sleep. In particularly advanced cases, it can lead to amputation. Right now, there are very few good options for treatment to slow its progression. As the Longevity Trial results show, it's also of great concern to those living with diabetes.

Even subjects who were not experiencing pain had higher levels of distress and depression around neuropathy—greater than that associated with any other diabetes complication. This finding was one that spurred Perkins' interest in the potential of corneal confocal microscopy. If clinicians were able to predict who would develop neuropathy, then more could be done to ensure it was better managed, and more people could avoid the worst impacts of this complication.

Currently, you can best test for early nerve damage in research studies using a biopsy of the skin. This is an effective technique, but not ideal. "It's just not so fun. I don't love the idea of people with diabetes getting skin biopsies every year," Perkins says. These procedures are painful and invasive, and not the ideal option just to find out if someone might be at risk. That's why the work being done on the cornea has elicited so much interest. "It turns out that the cornea of the eye is an adapted skin layer, and we can look with a high-powered microscope directly at these nerves. So, we're hoping to use this as a test to predict who is at risk of significant peripheral nerve injury."

Perkins' earnest desire to solve these puzzles—even if it's often at an earlier stage than more cautious investigators—has made him a popular figure on the academic debate stage. A unique aspect of the research world (and one of the more entertaining presentations at any conference), academic debates allow researchers to face off in something of a battle of the data to determine if their research actually holds up. Scientists, who are known for their sometimes-caustic responses to the work of their peers, rarely pull punches. For example, an entire Twitter feed exists solely to quote the often-devastating comments provided for peer-reviewed papers. You don't walk into a debate unless you feel confident in your science.

At the 2018 American Diabetes Association (ADA) Professional Conference, Perkins was invited to debate the merits of corneal confocal microscopy to an audience of health care professionals from around the world. His debate opponent, Dr. Robert Singleton from the University of Utah, feels confocal corneal microscopy simply doesn't work all that well, and that the current gold standard—those biopsies discussed earlier—is more reliable. He gives credit to Perkins for his work on the Toronto Clinical Scoring System and the impact that's had on the field, but when it comes to confocal corneal microscopy, he's just not sold on it.

"The ADA frequently tries to arrange debates over scientific issues that they think will be entertaining," says Singleton. "And I think that Bruce and I both entered into this debate or discussion in that spirit." In other words, he is a fan of Perkins' work, and though they have agreed to disagree on this subject, it made for a lively discourse.

It was an interesting debate, Perkins notes, completely willing to accept that Singleton raised legitimate issues with the project, but it's clear that it did not dissuade him from his belief that the process could have potential. "I'm not saying corneal confocal microscopy is the be-all-and-end-all. I'm just saying that the reality is that the current research environment in neuropathy sucks, and we have failure after failure. Part of that reason is that our tool for measuring it is too blunt and at too late a stage. We need a more sensitive tool. This one looks promising, so we should not abandon it."

He also knows that the patients he sees care less about the process and more about getting to the point where the issues they face are being managed. If a new drug or treatment is going into clinical trials, they want to know that the purpose meets their needs. "No one cares about the protein in their urine; no one cares whether their nerve conduction studies are 32 metres per second rather than 42 metres per second. They care whether they have pain in their feet, whether they're losing their toes and getting ulceration," he says.

This same premise is what drives Perkins' work in an even more controversial area of diabetes research—using Sodium Glucose Linked Transporter inhibitors (SGLTis) alongside insulin to treat type 1 diabetes. While a person with type 1 diabetes will always need to take insulin to survive, for years, there has been discussion of an adjunctive or add-on therapy that could help improve overall outcomes.

SGLT inhibitors are a class of drugs that help the kidneys clear sugar from the body, decreasing the reliance on insulin. This can help lower blood sugars, reduce weight, and even improve blood pressure—and as shown in the 2015 results of the ground-breaking EMPA REG trial—SGLT inhibitors can also improve cardiovascular outcomes. They are, in many ways, a game-changer for those living with type 2 diabetes.

For those with type 1 diabetes, SGLTis have proven more complicated. Perkins, who was in the audience when the EMPA REG results were announced, was immediately interested in how this could translate into better results for those living with type 1 diabetes. It felt auspicious that, as with the DCCT results that spurred his initial interest in diabetes complications, Toronto's Dr. Bernard Zinman was on stage again, presenting the EMPA REG results, which garnered a standing ovation from the crowd.

"We have these drugs that have an amazing impact on type 2 diabetes, on smoothing out and lowering blood sugar exposure," Perkins says. "And if they work so damn well in type 2, why the hell wouldn't we aggressively and quickly test them in type 1 where the need for therapies is so great? Even if they're not the perfect solution for type 1, we need solutions now."

His desire to move quickly is borne of his own experiences with the disease, but also the patients he sees in his clinical practice and the children with type 1 who are struggling with the condition. If something could improve the quality of life for those with type 1, he wants to find that *now*.

The problem with SGLT inhibitor treatments in type 1 is that they have been shown to increase the risk of a condition called diabetic ketoacidosis, or DKA, which is a build-up of acids—on top of higher sugar—in the blood when there is not enough insulin action. This condition, which is far more common in those with type 1 diabetes, is not only dangerous but potentially fatal if left untreated. While the risk of DKA is not high, it is still there, and at the time of my writing, is one of the reasons that the Food and Drug Administration (FDA) and Health Canada have not yet approved the use of SGLT inhibitor treatments for those with type 1 diabetes, though several other countries have approved this use.

This divide in the diabetes community about whether or not the benefits outweigh the risks when it comes to SGLT inhibitor treatments in type 1 diabetes is why Perkins finds himself on stage in yet another debate, this time at the 2019 ADA conference. The room is packed, and social media is buzzing as he sets about explaining why he thinks this work needs to happen. In the end, many in the audience are deterred, quite understandably, by the fear of DKA, but the majority still feel it's worth pursuing the option of SGLT inhibitor treatments.

Talking to Perkins both before and after the debate, he is steadfast in his commitment to the potential of this therapy. Even with all the advances in monitoring blood sugars and the improvements in insulin, he notes, A1C levels continue to worsen, especially in younger people. DKA is a real and valid concern, but he points out that even without SGLT inhibitor therapies, people with type 1 diabetes still develop DKA—about five in every one hundred patients will experience the condition in a given year. Regardless of the therapy being used, he feels health care professionals need to find better strategies for prevention.

"DKA is already a problem that we have to handle, and we don't do a great job of it," he says. "If we have someone who is using this medication, we've got to make sure they really understand how to identify ketoacidosis and how to test for it. For example, there's a blood or urine strip that can check for ketones—and they need to know how to manage it and what to do with their insulin. And I feel like we need to do a way better job of educating everyone with type 1 about this, whether or not someone is going to go on an SGLT inhibitor."

While these treatments have not yet been approved in North America, they have been in Europe and Japan, so experts are closely watching their progress there. Processes to use at the first sign of DKA, including the STICH protocol, or the Canadian contribution called the STOP-DKA protocol, have also been developed to help better educate those who are using an SGLTi on ways to avoid developing DKA.

Perkins agrees that for all his optimism about this treatment, there's still that level of uncertainty that can be nerve-wracking for both doctor and patient. There are some patients for whom SGLT inhibitor therapies would not be an option because they aren't great at managing their ketones or are already successfully achieving their targets on their own. The latter group might not need the additional complication of an extra therapy, yet Perkins sees it as a worthwhile option to consider for those who need it and feel confident in monitoring their health.

"The thing is, we've introduced really effective things in type 1 diabetes care that have had a huge risk of ketoacidosis before. We've done it. When [insulin] pumps were first evaluated in type 1, they were associated with a five- to seven-fold increased risk of ketoacidosis, so we could have said, 'You know what, forget it, it's too risky, keep on injections.'" he says. "But in my heart of hearts, I know that pump therapy has really transformed care for a lot of people. That's the tool, an insulin pump, that helps them get through their day and achieve their targets, so I'm glad that they have that available."

Perkins, who himself uses an insulin pump, notes that these devices have improved significantly with time and experience. They are much safer now than when they were first established, yet the risk of developing DKA in type 1 diabetes remains at five events per 100 people with type 1 diabetes annually.

"We've just got to work harder on managing type 1 diabetes safely," he says. "If a new therapy comes along that reduces A1C and has great effects on blood pressure and weight and possibly helps prevent cardiovascular events, we could say, 'Well, forget about it, because it's going to increase this already high risk of ketoacidosis,' and I think that's a perfectly good view.

"I think a lot of patients could just say, 'I'm glad you've offered this to me, but I'm not ready to take on that risk.' But many patients will say, 'Listen, I'm on top of this. I understand how to self-manage and to monitor for ketoacidosis, and I'm ready to take on these benefits from this medication. I'm grateful that I have more choices available to me to help manage my diabetes in the best way that I personally can.' We just need to make sure we trust that they're confident in managing their diabetes safely when adding such a medication."

It is with this optimism that Perkins and a team of other experts presented to the FDA in late 2019 to again argue for the approval of the drug as an adjunct or add-on therapy for those with type 1 diabetes. With all the new protocols in place and with the option of a low-dose treatment—which had shown efficacy without the increase in DKA seen at higher dose levels—the team was hopeful.

I was about to go on stage to moderate a panel in November 2019 when I received a text from a mutual friend of both Perkins and me, saying that the FDA committee had turned down the request for approval. "Bruce is going to be so upset," our friend wrote.

And he was. "Soul crushing," was how he put it when I followed up with him. While he understands, on some level, the fear of taking any risk, it's hard for him to understand the reticence when there is so much possibility in this area. He isn't sure if there is the appetite or funding for the large-scale clinical trials of low-dose SGLTis that would likely be needed to win eventual approval in the U.S. "As DKA is relatively rare, especially in clinical trial participants, a trial designed to examine this as an outcome needs to be enormous—especially if the goal is to demonstrate similar risks between the low-dose drug and the usual standard of care. Simply put, unlike in type 2 diabetes, it is very hard to study five, ten, twenty thousand people in a trial, because type 1 diabetes is so much less common than type 2 diabetes," he says.

Still, he admits that whatever the case, he will likely still be a part of the process as the next steps are determined. While the disappointment stings, the need to find better treatments remains.

It's easy to assume that much of Perkins' urge to develop new treatments and get them to patients quickly stems from the fact that he himself lives with type 1 diabetes. He has spoken often about the fear he initially felt that his diagnosis would hold him back. At just eighteen, when he was ready to start out on a life full of adventure, he was suddenly handed a diagnosis that changed everything.

Having interviewed many people living with type 1 diabetes over the years, including several who have gone on to work in diabetes research, there's a certain thread of overachievement that's woven into many of their lives. While some struggle to manage the condition, it's as though for others, the discipline it takes to live a healthy life with diabetes and the sheer will to thrive despite the difficulties spills over into everything they do.

Perhaps this is because many of those with type 1 diabetes are diagnosed in childhood when it is easier to form habits that shape a lifetime. Careful management of what they eat, constant monitoring of how activity affects their glucose levels, and the incredible vigilance needed for every aspect of their health can be exhausting and overwhelming, but it can also make someone even more driven to excel. NHL hockey star Max Domi has spoken frequently about how his diabetes fuels his athletic ability, and the list of highly accomplished celebrities and professional athletes living with the condition is extensive.

There is also the drive to help others living with diabetes, to tell people who are often very young when they are diagnosed that this disease is not easy, but it doesn't need to stop them. This is what inspired Beth Mitchell to take part in the Longevity Study, a time-intensive process involving hours of tests and invasive questions, but one she felt was important for those who were newly diagnosed with this disease. She volunteered, she says, because she *could*. "I thought, well, I can do this, and maybe they'll find something that will help treat it or find something that will say 'Oh, *this* is the key,' something that will help find a cure."

Whether Perkins and his team will find the links they are hoping to uncover remains to be seen. The third phase of the Longevity Study is being planned, and there is still much work to be done. The team at Perkins' lab has looked at many aspects of the results, including comparing them against those of a similar study done in the U.S. They've discovered that Canadians with type 1 diabetes have higher A1C levels than their American peers, yet much lower rates of cardiovascular disease. But some of the most important outcomes from this study have come through talking to the patients themselves.

As Perkins notes, when he started the project in 2012, he wanted to understand type 1 diabetes through the lens of those who have lived a lifetime with the condition. While the goal was to understand the factors that lead to complications, in the end, the project became more about the people they were studying. It was a far more rewarding and emotional journey than they had anticipated.

From the ninety-three-year-old participant who had lived with type 1 diabetes for eighty-two years to the "youngsters" in the study like Mitchell, the research team were charmed and inspired by the subjects of their work.

* * * * *

Leif Erik Lovblom is a biostatistician and PhD student in the Perkins Lab with a Master's degree in mathematics. When I ask to talk to him about his role in the lab for this book, he worries that his work as "the numbers guy" isn't as interesting as what the clinician-scientists are contributing. Yet, it is Lovblom, in his quiet, methodical way, who has collected and distilled all the data from the Longevity Study, the reams of numbers and statistics that have given proof to the theories and ideas the team put forward. It has also helped him find a way to use his skill with numbers to make a difference for those living with diabetes.

Lovblom, who himself lives with type 1 diabetes, had not been involved in health research before he came to work for Perkins, yet he's found his role in the lab to be a rewarding way to use mathematics to improve people's lives. His PhD thesis, conceived after several years of working with Perkins, looks at how to use statistical techniques to help understand the natural history of diabetes complications.

For him, the people who took part in the Longevity Study are at the heart of his work as he moves forward. "I learned there is a great diversity of experiences of type 1 diabetes," he says, noting the range of complications and individual challenges he saw in the data he compiled. He was also able to hear about these differences in the life stories shared by the participants.

There was, throughout, a unifying theme he found incredibly inspiring. "At diagnosis, which would have been in the 1960s and prior, many participants were told they would have kidney failure or blindness by the time they reached adulthood. I learned that people were able to overcome these negative outlooks and stereotypes, and ultimately live normal and healthy lives with diabetes."

This realization, and the understanding that to continue to thrive fifty years into a life with type 1 diabetes is possible, is exactly what Perkins set out to prove when he started his own research.

When asked if he does anything differently as a physician or a scientist because he also lives with type 1 diabetes, Perkins is always quick to say that his colleagues are just as likely to do the same things he does and to treat patients just as well as he would. He realizes there are specific individuals who want to see him because they think he will have some new insight that an endocrinologist without diabetes wouldn't have, but he's not sure that's true.

I press him on this point. Having known him several years and seen firsthand his interactions with the diabetes community, I'm not quite convinced that he doesn't bring a certain empathy to his work that someone without diabetes might not.

He thinks about this for a moment, then asks me if, given that, he should consider giving up research and work full time as a clinician. As a clinician-scientist, he can only see patients a day or two a week. Though he loves his medical practice, with so few hours available, the number of patients he can take on is relatively tiny. He worries about the lengthy waitlist for an appointment with him.

The first time Perkins asked me this question, years earlier, it left me a bit stunned that this prestigious scientist wanted *my* opinion on whether or not he should continue with science. Now, the question no longer surprises me. Whenever I mention the unique position he is in as an endocrinologist living with and treating people with type 1 diabetes, it seems to trigger a concern that he is somehow not giving enough to those who would benefit from his firsthand knowledge. It is, in its way, a quintessential Bruce Perkins quandary—called to do more research, but also wanting to encourage and support those who live with this disease, to ensure they live a life just as full as if they did not have diabetes. A life as full as his own.

In reality, Perkins will have far more impact and help far more people as a scientist than he ever could as simply a practicing endocrinologist. He already has.

His experience as a person living with diabetes colours his research and affects his clinical practice. He may insist that someone without diabetes would provide the same quality of treatment, perhaps even *better* treatment, and he could be right. But I believe his unique circumstances ensure the patients he *is* able to see have a physician who truly understands their frustrations and their fears—the very same qualities that drive and increase the impact of his research.

"I'm not sure it's really different," he says, "but I will tell you what I say to someone, for example, who has been admitted to hospital with new-onset type 1 diabetes in diabetic ketoacidosis. I will tell them first of all that it really sucks that they have diabetes and that I understand that, and that I wish they weren't dealing with this today. But the second thing is that no matter how terrible it seems, learning all the hundreds of tasks that someone with diabetes, unfortunately, needs to learn and get a hold of very quickly, they can still feel confident that they will be able to lead a life with diabetes that's as wonderful as a life *without* diabetes. These days we've got the kinds of insulin therapies, devices, and screening tests for early complications, and we have this wonderful framework to help someone reach their goals in their life, whether they have diabetes or not."

He pauses for a second and then continues. "I feel that other professionals in diabetes probably give that exact same message, and it probably comes off the exact same way, but for me when I say it, it's definitely an emotional one because I've been there, and I've felt it."

CHAPTER FOUR
Alberta and the Islet

When Bob Teskey was nineteen, he was found passed out in a snow-bank during a freezing Edmonton winter. Teskey had been walking through the University of Alberta campus when he was hit by an extreme hypoglycemia incident, losing consciousness and falling into the snow alongside the walkway. Had a fellow student not found him and gotten him help, Teskey might just have died in the snow that night.

Diagnosed with type 1 diabetes in 1961 at age fourteen, Teskey has a type of extreme hypoglycemia unawareness that is both rare and extremely dangerous. The majority of people with diabetes know when their blood sugar is going low and are able to treat the condition with fast-acting glucose tablets or a sugary drink. Unfortunately, Teskey is not able to feel the onset of a low-blood-sugar episode, and this has resulted in multiple near-death scares. While this did not curtail his successful completion of university and a career as a highly regarded lawyer, it did colour every aspect of his life.

Teskey and I meet at the Alberta Diabetes Institute on a sunny October day in 2019, and he fills me in on his history with the building. It was at the hospital next door where he spent his first few weeks after his diagnosis. Then he was in a ward full of veterans from both world wars, who took the young teen under their wing as he learned to inject insulin with a syringe by practicing on an orange.

He has a quiet matter-of-factness as he tells me about what must have been a traumatic diagnosis and some very frightening incidents brought on by his hypoglycemia unawareness. Yet perhaps it is his stoic nature that has helped him excel despite these challenging circumstances. Growing up at a time when glass syringes to administer insulin and urine testing strips to test blood sugar were the norm, when many saw diabetes as a life sentence, Teskey tried not to let it interfere with his goals. He ran several small businesses during high school and then enrolled in university upon graduation—a non-negotiable for his parents, diabetes or no.

"I was fortunate that my folks didn't try to limit me in what I could do by way of activities, so they accepted that if I wanted to go down a particular road, that was my choice," he says. "I know they worried, but they cut me a lot of slack. That was worth a lot over the course of my life because I learned then that you shouldn't treat diabetes as any kind of a limiting factor. You should treat it as a *complicating* factor, but not a limiting factor."

Teskey married a teacher, Hazel, in 1976, and they had two children. He had a busy career as a lawyer, travelling frequently and working on high-profile cases. He volunteered in the diabetes community when he could, and despite still dealing with incidents of hypoglycemia unawareness, he did not feel in any way restricted by his diagnosis. That changed in 1996 when he fell from the roof of his cottage, where he was making repairs. The fall was not caused by low blood sugar, but like many with diabetes, he had difficulty healing. The expected six weeks in a clamshell cast for his broken back escalated into six long and excruciating months as he slowly recovered.

Then, in a heart-wrenching twist of fate, Teskey and his wife were hit by a drunk driver just a year later, as they drove to the cottage on Thanksgiving weekend. Hazel was killed in the accident, and Teskey broke his leg and arm. He was suddenly a single parent and trying to heal from his injuries while mourning the loss of his wife.

On top of all this, his hypoglycemia unawareness was getting worse. "My kids put a baby monitor in my room so that they could listen for weird noises and activities, and it was becoming a much more limiting factor than it ever had before," he recalls. When he discussed it with his endocrinologist, there were few options. "There's very little that can be done. You can try to adjust your insulin a little bit, you try to have safety provisions in place, but at the end of the day, the advice and the help is fairly limited."

Though frustrated, Teskey had resigned himself to soldiering on as always when his endocrinologist called and asked if he would consider participating in a research study where he would receive an islet transplant. "My response, I remember it as clearly as it was yesterday, was, 'Just tell me where to turn up, and I'll be there.'"

Within your pancreas, there are groups of cells called beta cells, which produce insulin, and alpha cells, which produce glucagon. These groups, or clusters, are called islets. For people with type 1 diabetes, these cells have been largely destroyed, and the pancreas cannot make enough insulin. The procedure Teskey had signed up for would attempt to replace his broken islet cells with working ones from organ donors. He had no idea when he agreed to participate that he would be part of a discovery that would change the way the world looked at the possibility of a cure for type 1 diabetes.

* * * * *

Doctors James Shapiro and Ray Rajotte could not be more different in appearance or temperament. Shapiro, tall and reed-thin, is a soft-spoken, methodical Brit. Rajotte is shorter and stockier and exudes the warmth of the small-town Prairie boy he is. He laughs easily and will happily talk your ear off about the research being done in his province and the role Edmonton has played in changing the face of diabetes treatment worldwide. It is easy to see how the amiable and charming Rajotte has been able to turn the Alberta Diabetes Institute into a well-funded powerhouse of research excellence.

There would be much less for Rajotte to brag about without Shapiro's work to turn Rajotte's islet research program into an internationally-renowned success story. However, spending time with both men makes it hard not to recognize how much one needed the other.

Rajotte did not set out to be a diabetes researcher. Growing up in Wainwright, Alberta, he was interested in many different elements of medicine and science, deciding first to become an X-ray technician, and graduating from the program at the University of Alberta in 1965. It was a good job, but he wasn't content to just settle into it. Flipping through a magazine one day, a headline caught his eye: "Biomedical Engineer: The Career of the Future." He'd never heard of the profession, but he liked the sound of it.

The University of Alberta didn't have a biomedical engineering program at that time, so Rajotte was persuaded to sign up for the electrical engineering stream, with the promise that by the time he got through his first two years, there would be a biomedical designation. Two years later, there wasn't, but the school allowed him to take medical courses as his electives, and by the time he graduated, his degree was listed as biomedical engineering. He believes he was the first person from the university to graduate with that designation.

Continuing to work as an X-ray technician in the evenings and over the summer while he was in school, Rajotte also started to consider working in research. He landed a spot in the lab of Dr. George Bondar, a surgeon at the Edmonton General Hospital, who was also doing research on blood flow in tumours at the University of Alberta's Surgical Medical Research Institute. There wasn't much space available at the time, so Rajotte was left to work in an unused bathroom in the basement—his lab bench propped up over the urinals. It was an inauspicious start for the man who would one day lead the institute, and whose face, sculpted in bronze, is now hanging on the wall of the Alberta Diabetes Institute, which he helped to found.

While his first research program was interesting, Rajotte was eager to expand his knowledge and use his engineering skills. He convinced Dr. John Dosseter, an established Edmonton scientist, to take him on as a student, and he began work assisting Dosseter in cryopreserving kidneys. This was the project that would spark his future interest in islet transplantation, though, at the time, he saw it simply as an entry point into an area that seemed creative and useful. It was not, however, without its challenges.

"I thought, well, I'm going to start freezing kidneys. And we thought at the time we had to do rapid thawing," says Rajotte, who admits when he was first introduced to Dosseter's work, he wasn't even sure how to pronounce the word *cryobiology*, let alone do it. "I built these gadgets to perfuse the kidney, to cool them down to sub-zero temperatures, and then I used a microwave—and back then, you didn't go out and buy your microwave—so you had to build your own."

Because of his engineering background, Rajotte was able to figure out the technology to make his microwave, including a way to rotate the kidney so there wouldn't be hot spots. With that established, he froze the kidneys down to sub-zero temperatures of –200 degrees C. "I turned up the power, and it drew so much power, the lights went down, and all of a sudden, after 30 seconds, a big explosion—*boom*—and I opened the door, and there's kidney all over the place," he says, laughing now at what at the time seemed like an enormous miscalculation. It turned out that the cryoprotectant he had used on the kidneys had changed the properties of the organs. Instead of not absorbing energy, like most things do when frozen, they absorbed *a lot* of energy. And, well … boom.

Even with the initial problems, the work seemed promising. If you could freeze donated organs and then successfully thaw them, it would be much easier to manage organ donations. The project was notable, but it wasn't until 1970, when Dr. Paul Lacy from Washington University in St. Louis, Missouri, released a paper about the successful isolation and transplantation of those, that Rajotte found the work that would inform the rest of his career. "I said, that's interesting, they're small, maybe I should try to cryopreserve them," he recalls. He approached Dosseter, who encouraged him to try it, and who supervised his student's novel PhD project: *The successful cryopreservation of a cellular structure.*

Following that, Rajotte worked with some of the top islet scientists around the world. But after a few years, he returned to the University of Alberta to continue the research that now consumed him in the province that would always be home. There he was a member of the Department of Surgery, giving him access to some wonderful postdoctoral students. His first, Garth Warnock, would go on to have a pivotal role in the future of the Alberta islet program.

The research at the time was at the basic discovery level, done mostly in rats. Rajotte knew that in order to move the project forward into humans, he would need a clinical team of surgeons and endocrinologists, which he set about assembling.

One of the things you realize when spending time with Rajotte is that perhaps his greatest talent is in assembling the right people at the right time to move a project forward. Whether it be in building a research team or developing a fundraising plan to pay for said research, Rajotte has an amazing ability to bring all of the essential players together.

He is also eager to give credit. In the three hours we chat, Rajotte drops names faster than I can possibly follow. It feels like every mentor, student, or donor who has ever contributed to his programs is mentioned in some way. It's hard not to like that about him, though there's no way to include that exhaustive list of notable people in this chapter. Even with all he has achieved, Rajotte seems compelled to remind me there's no way he could have accomplished any of it alone.

With the beginnings of a clinical team in place, Rajotte was able to move the islet research project from rats into larger mammals and then into humans. They used donated pancreases to practice isolating human islets using the techniques they had developed in animals. Knowing they would need to better understand how to work with the human immune system for any transplant work to be successful, Rajotte sent Warnock to study immunology at Oxford.

Then Rajotte brought in Norm Kneteman, whom he warmly refers to as "a local boy from Edson." Kneteman was able to help the team make the leap from isolating islets to cryopreserving them. "What we had learned in the rats, we were able to extrapolate that from humans. And eventually, that became important when we carried out Canada's first islet transplant," Rajotte says.

From there, Kneteman spent time in St. Louis learning more about transplantation, and Rajotte began to think this project finally had legs. "Now I've started my puzzle," he remembers. "We've got basic scientists who can isolate human islets, and we wanted to start clinical trials."

To move their lab work into human subjects, they needed an endocrinologist. Rajotte enlisted Dr. Edmond "Eddie" Ryan, who had just moved to Edmonton from Miami. Ryan identified some candidates that would be good options for the clinical trial. They wanted those who had type 1 diabetes but who were also in need of a kidney transplant. Because of the need to put the patient on immunosuppressants after a transplant, it made more sense to test a new procedure on someone who was already going to require those drugs to support the more established transplant.

With all of this in place, in 1989, the team carried out Canada's first islet transplant. The transplant, while a major step forward, was not entirely a success. The matching process back then was not as strong, and the patient developed cytomegalovirus (CMV), a strain of the herpes virus, likely because the donor was unknowingly infected. The team also learned through this process that the antirejection drugs and steroids being used to protect the kidney transplant were toxic to the islets. While the patient recovered from the infection and had good islet function for a time, the researchers knew they had more work to do.

Another transplant patient followed, who also developed CMV. The process didn't really take, so when they tried a third time, they increased the number of islets. In that case, the patient was insulin independent for almost three years and still had good blood sugar control more than 15 years later. It was an exciting breakthrough, Rajotte notes, but the process was still in its infancy.

They were also in need of funding. While there was some support from health charities and the government, this type of research is extremely expensive. Rajotte spent much of his time talking to potential donors, and it was through these discussions that the Alberta Diabetes Foundation (ADF) was formed in 1989. Having a provincial organization dedicated to supporting the work being done in the province—in particular the islet research program—meant the team would have ongoing financial support. Thirty years later, the ADF continues to be an enormous resource for the province's diabetes research programs.

As the islet transplant program continued to grow and other re-search centres around the world started their own clinical trials of the process, it was clear that there was potential. Yet only about ten per-cent of those who received a transplant became insulin independent, even for a short time. For a very difficult and expensive procedure, those weren't great numbers.

So, from 1989 to 1999, the team worked on refining the process. Throughout that time, they did joint islet-kidney transplants because of the ethics of giving someone immunosuppressants for islet trans-plants alone when there was little evidence the procedure worked. Rajotte credits Eddie Ryan for suggesting they try an islet-alone transplant, using antirejection drugs they felt would be less toxic. Ra-jotte agreed, but he knew that to do that successfully, they would need to expand the team. "Back then, it was tough to recruit people, but I always found people that had family ties here," he says.

Enter Gregory Korbutt, another of Rajotte's trainees, who he sent from Edmonton to Brussels to learn how to manipulate the cells so they would reject less quickly. "I was building a team of not only transplant surgeons," Rajotte says. "But also immunologists, to try and figure out this whole process of how do we make the islets work better using different antirejection drugs."

The key figure, though, was arguably Dr. James Shapiro. The tall, imposing Brit is as stoic as Rajotte is gregarious. From Newcastle upon Tyne in England, he had approached Norm Kneteman about doing a transplant fellowship with him in Alberta.

In his neat, sunny office at the University of Alberta in the fall of 2019, Shapiro explains that in England, he'd been working on a thesis on islet transplantation and the rat. Then he stands to pull the thick, imposing bound book containing the project off his shelf. Hand-typed, it's the sort of time capsule of the work that will one day likely be in a museum.

When Shapiro arrived in Edmonton, he became the missing link that helped turn the islet transplant program there into the worldwide success story it is today. After finishing his PhD, Shapiro had consid-ered leaving to follow his interest in pancreas transplant, but Rajotte convinced him to stay, promoting him to clinical director. By then, Rajotte was the director of the Surgical Medical Research Institute, where the islet work was being done, and he was eager to have Shapiro continue with the progress he was making.

"When I came, they'd had this attempt to do a handful of islet transplant patients back in the late 1980s and early 1990s, and the program really generated a lot of interest to start with, but then it failed," Shapiro explains, noting that in the five years he'd been working on his PhD in Edmonton, there hadn't been any human transplants attempted. There was a lot of work being done on making islets, but that also meant a lot of barriers and issues.

"They asked me if I would run that program because I'd researched islet transplant. I was doing a PhD in islet transplant," Shapiro says. "I was an expert in clinical surgery and clinical transplantation, and an expert in the antirejection drugs, so it seemed a natural fit for everybody if I, as a transplant surgeon, would come and run this program. So I said yes, but I'd only do it on the condition that I could dramatically change things around, because when I looked at the literature, there had been 300-odd attempts to do islet transplants in patients—286 to be exact—and virtually none of them worked. None of them were working after the first year or so, and if they were working, it was very minimal."

At this point in the conversation, Shapiro pulls out another thick volume from his shelf—this one containing his PhD work in Alberta. While he no longer had to hand-type the document, the work that went into it was nothing short of remarkable. It was in these pages that he outlined the process that would become the Edmonton Protocol.

Much had changed since the first in-human trials in 1989, and the research team was now able to isolate more viable islets. They knew they needed more of them—a minimum of 5,000 to 10,000 islets per kilogram of body weight—and the antirejection drugs were better. There was also more mutual understanding and talent on the team.

Shapiro enlisted a PhD student named Jonathan Lakey, who was skilled at isolating human islets. The pair travelled to two of the major research centers studying islet transplants internationally—in Miami, Florida, and Giessen, Germany—to try and improve on the techniques for making islets that they were using in Alberta at the time. Returning to Edmonton with their newfound knowledge, the pair worked with the islet team to prepare for their next round of in-human clinical trials.

This time, the process was a success. "On March the 11th, 1999, we had a patient taken down to the X-ray department. His name was Byron, and he had long-standing diabetes for about 30 to 40 years," Shapiro explains.

Like Bob Teskey, Byron had dangerous lows in his blood sugars that he was unable to control despite intensive insulin therapy. Shapiro and the team had a procedure they hoped would help. "We infused islet cells into the liver via a nonsurgical approach. The X-ray doctors passed a little tube in through the skin and in through the liver, and into the vein going up to the liver, which is called the portal vein. We infused the islet cells up into the liver where they nested, they formed a new blood supply, and his insulin requirements dropped by at least half within days of the infusion," Shapiro says of that first transplant. "We gave him a second infusion, and after that, he was completely free of insulin."

This was around the time that Teskey had received the call from his endocrinologist, asking if he wanted to take part in a research study. He had readily agreed, even before meeting with Shapiro to discuss the process, but once the two had talked—and it was determined that Teskey was a good candidate for the procedure—he became patient number four.

"The first transplant went really quite smoothly, and the next day my insulin requirements had dropped by half just overnight," Teskey recalls. While he still had to take some insulin, the reduction had an immediate—and very positive—impact on his life. The process was also much less invasive than many of the previous transplant procedures, and Teskey was back at work the following day.

Six weeks later, Shapiro called to ask if Teskey would like a second transplant, adding more cells to shore up the first graft, to which

Teskey readily agreed. This procedure was less successful, however. "It didn't really move the needle much," Teskey recalls of his insulin needs. In August, a third transplant was so successful that he was even off insulin for a time, having normal A1C levels for four years.

Teskey was one of seven successful transplants performed using the process that Shapiro had perfected. It was a breakthrough unlike any other, and the team quickly wrote a paper outlining the technique and these seemingly incredible results.

The New England Journal of Medicine published the manuscript in July 2000, and the world took notice. The University of Alberta and the research team members were besieged by media requests about this fantastic new process called the Edmonton Protocol, which could allow someone who needed regular insulin injections in order to survive to no longer have to take them at all. Even then-President Bill Clinton acknowledged the researchers and this remarkable result in one of his regular press briefings.

Could it be possible that these doctors and scientists working in Alberta had really figured out how to cure type 1 diabetes?

Well, sort of.

A physician friend who does not work in diabetes recently interrupted me as I was telling him about the Edmonton Protocol. "But I thought that doesn't work," he said, confused. "That's why we're not doing it for people."

He was a bit mixed up, which is understandable because islet cell transplants are tricky to explain. While the Edmonton Protocol was a resounding success and Shapiro notes that more than forty health centres worldwide now do the procedure—with more than two thousand having been done since 1999—it's neither easy nor common.

That's because, while it works extremely well in some people, there are many complex factors that inhibit the ability to do islet transplants. There aren't enough islet cells available, to name one very big barrier.

Dr. Peter Senior is one of those magnanimous people that you can't help but like. An affable Brit, he found his way to the Alberta Diabetes Institute the same way many do—he wanted to learn how to do islet transplants. An endocrinologist and scientist who has become a beloved leader in the Canadian diabetes community, he jokes that he must be a very slow learner because almost twenty years after arriving in Edmonton, he's still there.

Senior decided to pursue his career in the city because once he realized the potential for islet transplants and the incredible impact they could have on the lives of people with diabetes, it was hard to leave the research behind. The process, which has been refined since the initial few transplants, *is* somewhat magical.

"We take pancreases from donors who died, and they're donating all of their organs potentially for transplantation. But rather than taking the whole pancreas and putting it into another person, which would be a big, big surgery with significant risks, we can actually take the organ that's maybe 4 ounces, or 100 grams, process it with quite a lot of hard work to extract the cells which make insulin, and that ends up being less than a teaspoonful," Senior explains.

"Those can then be infused into a vein that drains into the liver. The islets then set up home in the recipient's liver, and they will make insulin to keep the blood sugar rock steady. It's a bit like setting cruise control on your blood glucose levels because the islets will make more insulin when the sugars are high and turn off when the sugars are normal. So, we can restore stable blood glucose levels predictability, and most importantly, for the patients we treat, we abolish bad hypoglycemia, and that's a huge step forward for many of our patients."

But, again, donor islets are hard to come by. Someone has to die and be registered as an organ donor. They also have to have healthy islets. They can't have diabetes or other related health conditions. Rajotte estimates there are 400 to 500 organs available each year, but not all of them end up in islet programs. With approximately 300,000 Canadians living with type 1 diabetes, that's just a drop in a very large bucket. For now, the procedure has mainly been limited to those who have the greatest difficulty in managing their diabetes—those with hypoglycemia unawareness—as they are most likely to see the biggest benefits from receiving a transplant.

"There will never be enough organ donors in the world to treat all the people, so we need to get alternative sources of cells and work out how to transplant them safely," explains Senior. This has led researchers, including Shapiro, to look at options like stem cells, to figure out ways to manage the supply and demand issue.

While the transplants are successful when the islets are available to make them possible, they have other limitations. The antirejection drugs needed to ensure the transplant takes can be very hard on the body. Some people complain of mouth sores or other ailments, and some are so bothered by the drugs that they go off them completely and let the transplanted islets die off because it's too much to manage the side effects. This is one reason children are not eligible for islet transplants under the current process—keeping them on antirejection drugs for life could be entirely too hard on their bodies.

In addition, while the transplanted cells seem to provide a period of insulin independence, they slowly stop working. This means that someone who has a transplant and is off insulin for several years may have to return to using insulin as the transplants wane. In the early days of the treatment, this was especially common.

Bob Teskey's first transplants started to fail after about four years. "While apparently, I was still producing some insulin on the basis of the lab test, for all intents and purposes, from about 2004 until 2012, I was back on pretty much a full dose of insulin, and with all of the side effects, including all of the lows," Teskey says.

He had remarried in 2003, and his new wife, a dietitian, became very good at predicting when a low was coming on, which was helpful. He'd also started to develop heart problems, however, another common complication of diabetes. Still, when Shapiro approached him in 2013 about another islet transplant, this time using the more refined techniques that had developed since his first procedure, Teskey was game.

Once they had determined that his heart and kidney issues would not be a problem, he was ready to go. "By 2013, the process was much more complex, but in any event, I had one transplant then, and a follow-up transplant because they thought they could get better function," Teskey says. Because his 1999 transplant was from two donors,

Teskey now has islets from six donors in his system, which he thinks likely makes him the person with the largest number of islet donors in the world today.

"The result of the 2013 transplant has been interesting," he says. "I was only off insulin for a relatively short period of time, but since then, and continuing to the present time, I've been on a much-reduced intake of insulin, and the overall control has been absolutely amazing. What the transplant does is give you a stability that you just never see in type 1."

For someone with type 1 diabetes, it is not uncommon for blood sugars to veer into the 20s or dip into the low 4s. This is no longer an issue for Teskey.

"My blood sugars are always in a very constant range. And the real proof of the pudding is that when I had significant problems with my kidneys this past year, I had an A1C at one point of 5.6. Well, 5.5 is kind of the normal person on the street, so 5.6 is almost unheard of for an insulin-dependent diabetic. And even now, when they've encouraged me to not be so tightly controlled because they worry about the lows, it's around 6 or 6.2. So, on one level, you could view the 2013 transplant as something of a failure because I didn't get off insulin at all, but for me, it's been a giant success because it's given me the stability that is unheard of. I still have to take some insulin, I still have some trouble with lows, but the stability is remarkable."

This is the sort of result Senior tends to herald. When people talk about why someone would want to bother with an islet transplant, which may need to be re-done a few years later, instead of simply using one of the many technologies now available, he points out that the transplants confer some very positive results.

Blood sugar levels seem to stabilize greatly, even after the person goes back on insulin, which for those with hypoglycemia unawareness—the majority of those eligible for a transplant—can be life-changing. It can also help to reduce the risk of the many complications of diabetes, which are often the result of recurrent high or low blood sugars. Senior also knows that, even if it's only for a few years, that freedom is a critical period. As the technologies improve and the ability to make islets in the lab becomes more of a reality, he thinks many people would opt for a transplant over a closed loop or artificial pancreas system.

"Wearing a device that you have to have stuck onto you, that you have to tend and look after and fill with insulin and not get bumped off and all those things, that's not what most of my patients think of as the cure," he says. "They would like to go away and have surgery or get an injection, and then walk away and forget about that disease."

Islet transplants aren't there yet, but things are getting better. "I see the Edmonton Protocol and the islet cell transplant as a very successful experiment," says Shapiro, "But I don't see it as a real cure in the long term for patients with diabetes. But what it has done for us, it's absolutely in black and white proven that if you inject cells that make regulated insulin in patients, and the cells survive, you can basically cure the disease."

Shapiro and Senior have both taken their research into the realm of stem cells, hoping to find an unlimited source of islets that the body won't reject. Rajotte, meanwhile, has thrown himself into the work of supporting and funding it all.

After twenty-five years of leading the Surgical Medical Research Institute, the unit has been renamed for him—the Ray Rajotte Surgical Medical Research Institute. He has also put his considerable charm and talent at team building to use to build the Alberta Diabetes Institute (ADI). The ADI, which brings together diabetes research teams from across the province, is no longer just about islets, though they most certainly continue to lead the way. Rajotte helped raise more than $45 million to build a state-of-the-art facility, the one where the bust of his face now graces the lobby, and they have since added a stem cell GMP facility that took another $35 million to build.

He is incredibly proud of the work that has come out of his home province and the team of top-notch scientists and clinicians who have found their way to Alberta and the ADI because of the work of the Edmonton Protocol. This native of Wainwright, Alberta, who started out doing science in a bathroom in the basement, has left an incredible legacy. As Rajotte nears full retirement, whatever that may look like, the ADI's roster of top scientists continues to build on the foundation he has laid.

Shapiro shows no signs of slowing down. He is running multiple clinical trials trying to find a way to make islet transplants more practical. He has won many awards and honours for his work in the field, but he doesn't like to think much about what he's done. "I always look forward, not back," he tells me, motioning to the many framed awards sitting on his shelves, not yet hung.

He notes that many of the awards and medals he has been given for his accomplishments are at home in his sock drawer. He is solely focused on what he can do to improve outcomes for the patients he sees in his clinics, who may have had their lives made better by his work on the Edmonton Protocol, but who are still not cured. "I saw opportunities, and I see faults with it, and I see how it can be improved, and that's what I dedicate my life to now—how to make things better. I wouldn't say I'm ever proud of what I've done. I'd say I'm proud of what's yet to come."

CHAPTER FIVE

Building a Better Islet

When Dr. Cristina Nostro arrived in New York City from Manchester, England, to begin her postdoctoral studies, she only had two suitcases and an incredible drive to learn everything she could about stem cells.

Raised in Calabria, Italy, Nostro was studying stem cells in the blood as a PhD student in Manchester when Dr. Gordon Keller visited the city to give a talk. Keller, originally from Saskatoon, is considered a pioneer in the study of stem cells. His work looking at mouse stem cells to model blood development was world-leading, and Nostro was intrigued by the progress he was making in this relatively new area of research.

When she started to consider postdoctoral studies, Keller's lab was at the top of her list. She interviewed with him at the Black Family Stem Cell Institute at the Icahn School of Medicine at Mount Sinai in New York in 2003 and knew instantly this was the right fit. "I had done tours of labs in Europe and the U.S., and when I went there, I knew that I wanted to work there. The things they were doing were fascinating." Nostro jokes that she bugged Keller until finally, in May of 2004, he hired her to work in his lab.

When just a few years later, in 2006, Keller was tapped to run the stem cell program at the University Health Network in Toronto, Nostro went with him. Now, she runs her own lab at the McEwen Stem Cell Institute in that city. She has more than proven that Keller made the right choice in hiring her. She is leading a research team that is trying to solve the enormous challenge of how to increase the supply of human pancreatic islets needed to support the number of people with diabetes who could benefit from a transplant. As there are far too few donor islets available, Nostro is determined to use stem cells to make up the gap.

Stem cells were discovered by Drs. James Till and Ernest McCulloch in Toronto in 1961. Like many of the world's most exciting scientific advances, the finding was a happy accident. The pair stumbled upon the cells while working on a cancer research project involving radiation and mice. They found a type of cell in the bone marrow that was able to replace parts of the immune system that was destroyed during radiation. Since then, stem cells have been found in many parts of the body.

A unique type of stem cell is described as "pluripotent." These cells are remarkable for their potential. In the embryonic stage of life, they are like a blank canvas that, as an organism forms, take on specific roles and can make any part of the body. So, a pluripotent stem cell can mature to become a liver cell or a heart cell, or as in Nostro's work, a beta cell.

Since Till and McCulluch's discovery, scientists have been looking for ways to use stem cells to replace the cells in our body which are broken or defective in some way. There have been advances in the cancer field, with multipotent stem cells being used successfully in the treatments for leukemia and several other forms of the disease. However, despite the incredible potential and the myriad of not-so-reputable companies offering to cure everything from arthritis to autism using stem cells, so far the science remains mostly in the early stages.

While stem cells offer the possibility of new ways to treat disease, they are by no means a simple solution. Stem cells are living cells, which make them very different than traditional medications or vaccines. Think of it this way: I have an allergy to penicillin. If I take penicillin, I break out in hives. While frustrating and uncomfortable, once the drug leaves my system, the hives go away. Not so with stem cells. Once you inject cells into the body, they are there to stay.

But even before these cells can be injected into a person, there is a long process of making sure scientists are able to make the right type of cell for the right problem. Stem cells have the amazing potential to develop into any cell in our body but coaxing them into becoming exclusively the cells we want them to be is a complex process that scientists are still grappling with. And the consequences of getting this wrong are significant.

When stem cells develop in unintended ways, they not only fail to treat the issue they were meant to, but their growth can also result in something called a teratoma. I don't suggest googling the term, as the images you will find are stomach-turning. These masses of cells can actually develop into a form of cancer, or they can result in all sorts of strange physiological mash-ups, like a tooth growing in your pancreas. This is, as you can imagine, a great fear of those who work in the field.

However, as more and more projects move towards clinical trials that will determine if stem cells are safe and effective in humans, scientists like Nostro are hoping to see their lab-grown cells one day saving lives. "We have to do better than what we have right now in the clinic—which is insulin. People know that insulin is not ideal, but we know it's safe." When working with stem cells, there is still much that needs to be learned. "We have to be able to provide a product that is absolutely safe. We need to demonstrate that the cells will not turn into a tumour and that they will respond and produce insulin correctly."

Building a beta cell is also no easy task. Dr. Bruce Verchere, the director of the BC Diabetes Research Network and a scientist at the BC Children's Hospital, has spent more than twenty years studying beta cells. For Verchere, the idea of being able to grow beta cells in the lab that could then effectively be transferred into humans is intriguing. Like many who saw the success of the Edmonton Protocol and then the great disappointment that those with diabetes felt when they realized there simply aren't enough donor islets (the clusters of beta and alpha cells found in our pancreas), Verchere thinks stem cells could provide a solution.

However, given how precise and perfect the beta cells in a person without diabetes are, creating a version in the lab is more than a simple challenge. "There's about a billion of these cells that reside in our pancreas. In people with type 1 diabetes, those cells are mostly lost or so dysfunctional that patients need to take insulin because there's no insulin production. When they take insulin, they're making their best guess as to what their insulin needs are," Verchere says. For people without diabetes, there is no guesswork. "The beta cell really does that job quite exquisitely in your body. It senses the blood glucose level, and it releases just the right amount of insulin so that when your glucose goes up after a meal, insulin comes out of the beta cell and takes that glucose out of the blood and into tissue. And when glucose goes down, you don't want insulin in the blood anymore. That's what gives you lows, and so the beta cell turns off. And it's really this precise minute-to-minute, maybe even second-to-second regulation of insulin secretion."

Creating a lab-grown version of these beta cells has shown promise, but scientists admit they're just not there—yet. "We haven't generated the equivalent of the adult human beta cell in vitro [in the lab] from human pluripotent stem cells," Nostro explains. "We're very close. We can make cells that express and produce insulin and can release insulin, but we haven't really reproduced the full mature beta cell." She wonders, however, if being close enough is going to be, well, *enough*.

"I think the question we have to ask ourselves is, do we really need to have a perfect beta cell, or can we actually work with something that is slightly imperfect, but once it's transplanted into a human being, is able to function and normalize glycemia? I think potentially, we might already have something like that," she says, noting that an increasing number of research teams are starting to move toward clinical trials.

Scientists have already shown in other organ systems that immature cells are able to reach their full potential after transplantation, and this is because the other cells in the body help provide support and biological cues that assist the cells in maturing.

Nostro and her colleague in Toronto, Dr. Sara Vasconcelos, are using these examples to look into how to create this more nurturing environment for the cells. "If you transplant an organ like a liver or lung or a heart, the very first thing a surgeon would do is reconnect all the vessels that will connect the organ to the vasculature [blood system] in order for the organ to be nourished. When you transplant islets, you're essentially injecting them into the portal vein so that the islets will then seed into the liver," Nostro explains. "There is no real connection to the vasculature in the beginning, so what we are trying to do is improve the early vascularization." This process, she says, will provide the essential nourishment to the cells immediately, ensuring they don't start to die off. Instead, they will have access to the factors needed to help them mature.

If those cells are able to survive and function when implanted into humans, it could be a game-changer for people living with diabetes. Similar to those with diabetes who receive islet transplants, a patient who receives a stem cell transplant could potentially be free of having to monitor glucose levels and give insulin injections. The lab-derived beta cells would be able to monitor insulin levels and react just like healthy beta cells do in people without diabetes.

However, there are more considerations than just making a version that works and can survive. In type 1 diabetes, it is believed that the autoimmune system malfunctions and kills off the beta cells in the pancreas. What will stop that from happening again? And even if the immune system doesn't kill off the cells for that reason, how do we get it to accept a foreign substance into our bodies without simply rejecting this substance the way it fights off a virus?

In other transplant situations, like when a person receives a donor kidney or liver, they must take powerful anti-rejection drugs to keep the body from doing just that. These drugs often come with side effects that can run from unpleasant to intolerable. With type 1 diabetes often being diagnosed in young children, it would be a challenge for them to remain on these drugs throughout their lifetime.

Nostro thinks figuring out how to keep the body from rejecting the lab-derived cells is almost a bigger piece of the puzzle than actually making the cells themselves. "One way to do this would be to transplant the cells in an immuno-protective device. The first clinical trials have used such a device, and at the moment, we are trying to implement new devices that will protect the cells from being destroyed by the immune system."

One of these first-in-human trials of encapsulated cells derived from stem cells is being supported by research done in the lab of Dr. Timothy Kieffer at the University of British Columbia. The project takes human pluripotent stem cells—those that are at the stage when they have the potential to turn into any type of cell in the body— and puts them through a process called differentiation, which involves changing them from one cell type to another, so they develop into what are called "pancreatic progenitor cells."

"These cells are not yet mature insulin-producing cells, but they're kind of committed to that lineage," Kieffer explains. Since the goal is to turn them into cells from the pancreas, this kind of commitment means that while they are not yet fully mature beta cells, they can no longer become the cells of other organs such as the heart. Limiting the number of other cell types they can become is necessary for safety.

Once these cells have been differentiated into pancreatic progenitor cells, Kieffer explains, they can be put into a small device, a recent version of which he describes as resembling a teabag. "The idea is that the cells go into the device, the device is sealed, and then it's implanted under the skin of the patient."

This "teabag" ensures that the cells contained within it are protected from the immune system, which could otherwise react to the foreign cells and attack them. The pores of the "teabag" allow important nutrients to get in and feed the cells while the insulin is able to get out. Once the cells mature, a process that takes several months, they turn into insulin-producing beta cells.

It was in Kieffer's lab that the initial basic science showed that this type of transplant solution was possible—in mice. While a significant breakthrough, there is a running joke in the diabetes research community that this is a very good time to be a mouse with diabetes, as there are no shortage of cures.

While mice are often used in research because they possess very similar physiology to humans, what acts as a cure in them does not always translate into larger mammals. There are many reasons for this, among them that human bodies are much more complex than mice. And mice are often bred specifically to test a certain question—they may be bred without one gene or cell type in order to see if removing these can help decrease their risk of getting diabetes. This goes a long way to helping scientists understand what these genes or cells do and the role they play in disease, but it is not a simple way to find a cure in humans.

When I first started covering science, I would go to research presentations and listen to someone talk about how they removed gene X or Y from a mouse and how the mouse no longer grew obese or developed diabetes. Well, I thought, problem solved! Why aren't we doing that in people? It did not take me long to realize that if you take out X gene, you can cure a mouse of diabetes, but if you remove that same gene from a human, you may cure their diabetes, but you might also kill them. Or just make a mess of their cellular makeup and cause all sorts of other damage.

Other times, the funding is simply not available to take a promising discovery into larger trials. This is referred to in scientific circles as "the research valley of death." There is good evidence that something could be effective, but there's just not enough there for an investor or government funding agency to provide the millions—if not billions—of dollars needed to find out if it actually works and to make sure it doesn't cause more harm than good.

That Kieffer's discovery has gotten into human trials at all is a testament to the quality of his science and the potential that it shows. "I was very excited to see that industry was getting behind this and actually putting in the resources that are necessary to get it into testing in patients," he says.

Part of making this investment work will be ensuring that the process is scalable.

With her shock of fuchsia hair and her warm, infectious laugh, Priye Iworima makes a strong first impression. Iworima, originally from Port Harcourt in Nigeria, is a graduate student in Kieffer's lab when I meet her. Her role involves not only working to develop insulin-producing cells from stem cells but also to make sure that there is the ability to make the necessary amount of them.

Creating enough functional cells for treating diabetes in mice is difficult enough, but in order for any of this to be truly successful, there must be the ability to generate millions of these cells that can be used in transplants. "We're trying to produce a product that could be used as a replacement cell therapy for patients living with type 1 diabetes," she explains. "We really want to make sure that all the basic science we're doing to manufacture those cells means we can make a large enough number that could be used for the population."

Iworima talks about the complex stem cell science she does with an enthusiasm that is hard to contain. It is her role to help ensure the processes developed in the lab can be done on a scale that would meet the needs of patients. "The impact we could potentially make with the work that we're doing in the lab is in generating these cells that could be maturing and secreting insulin in a regulated manner, and actually looking at the process and making it scalable. It is amazing to be able to touch even one person's life, but there are millions of people who are affected with diabetes, so I just absolutely love the work."

For Alberta's Dr. James Shapiro, whose work on the Edmonton Protocol proved that islet transplants could be successful, any of these ideas could be the missing link to creating an unlimited supply of islets. Of the many projects Shapiro is currently working on, stem cells are at the heart of several. "Cures happen in steps," he says. "They're iterative. What you learn in one area helps you in another. We're getting closer and closer. And I really feel that there's a bit of a crescendo happening now, and the big crescendo for me is the stem cells."

Shapiro is understandably proud of what has been achieved already, but his research is now focused on how to make the process accessible to even more people. "I think we showed with the Edmonton Protocol that cell transplant has the potential to cure patients of diabetes. You give someone cells, they don't need insulin anymore, they have fantastic sugar control," he says.

However, he knows it's far from a cure in its current state.

That's why Shapiro's basic science work is now focussed on solving the limiting factors with transplants. One such project takes the blood of patients with diabetes and winds the cells back in time as if they were back in the embryo. This process is called reprogramming and generates IPS or inducible pluripotent stem cells. "We take those IPS cells from patients' own cells, and then we can wind them forward with the protocols that have been established by other scientists in Canada, including Tim Kieffer in Vancouver. Then we can turn those IPS cells into islet-like cells," he explains. "So now we have human islets basically, that make human insulin, and they're the patient's own, so they wouldn't be rejected by the immune system."

Shapiro considers the work of Nostro and Kieffer to be amongst the best in the world. "I think the embryonic stem cell and the IPS cell technology are absolutely the frontier of where Canada can lead. Canadian scientists have made the biggest contributions to the science and understanding of that already," he says. "Tim is an absolutely brilliant scientist; he's made so many prime discoveries in so many areas of diabetes that have been transformative. And it's basically his work that we're trying to copy on to take forward into patients."

Studying and understanding human islets is at the heart of all of these projects, and one of the reasons Canada's research teams are able to do the work they do is because of a program run by a soft-spoken, affable scientist at the Alberta Diabetes Institute (ADI). Dr. Patrick MacDonald had a number of options when it came to deciding where we would do his research, and he chose the University of Alberta and the ADI, he says, because of the potential of what he could accomplish working there.

He has more than lived up to that potential. MacDonald's Islet-Core program, which provides human islet and pancreas tissue for scientific research, is now one of the largest in the world. The project came about through discussions with Shapiro and his team. MacDonald and others studying cell physiology would benefit greatly from having human cells to use in their research; however, getting access to human tissues can be quite difficult and often depends on the availability of 'unused' islets from clinical transplant programs. The islet transplant program at the ADI had a great deal of unused donor organs, and MacDonald saw an opportunity. If these donated organs could not be used directly for transplantation, perhaps they could be used to help better understand diabetes at a cellular level, in developing treatments and, at some point, even a cure.

"I come from a very basic side of things, but we want to do work that is relevant to people," he explains. "We want to study these cells to better understand how insulin and other hormones are made. The clinical group was turning down about 120 organs a year that they couldn't use for various reasons. Maybe the donor had diabetes, maybe it was just not a good match for a recipient, but these are the kind of things we really want to study. We can learn so much from studying the islets of people with diabetes."

Now when a donor pancreas is not viable for a transplant, and all of the consents have been received from the donor family, MacDonald and his team ensure that the organ is used for appropriate academic research. The program launched in 2010, and their lab, on the fifth floor of the ADI, does islet isolations from human donors specifically for research purposes. "The program has since grown quite a lot. We provide more human islets for research than any other group in the world now," he explains. "We supply tissue to about 110 different groups around the world for basic science study of human islet biology, which touches on genetics and regenerative medicine and metabolism, cell biology, transplantation, all kinds of things."

MacDonald is proud of what the program has accomplished. "It puts us in a position where we can impact how human islet research is done," he says. "An obvious example is stem cells being turned into beta cells or islet cells for transplants. If you're going to do that, you really need to know what standard it is you need to achieve, and you have to understand what the gold standard is, what it is you're aiming for." Being able to study human tissue, both healthy or with diabetes, allows for that in a way that could not be achieved in animal models.

"There's still a lot we don't understand about how human islets work, and that's really what we're trying to figure out," MacDonald says. For example, insulin production varies greatly from person to person. Does that mean that those looking to create islets or beta cells in the lab need to create cells that are unique to each person? Or will finding one that works well enough in the majority of people be good enough? These are among the questions scientists using tissue provided by MacDonald's program hope to answer.

Sitting in her office in Toronto's MaRS Discovery Centre, one of Canada's research and technology hubs, Nostro sips a cappuccino as she considers where the field is now. Stem cells have come a long way in a short time. They were discovered in the 1960s, started to be a part of the broader research field in the 1990s, and now they are on the cusp of many significant breakthroughs. But there is still much work to be done.

Nostro became a Canadian citizen in 2019. She feels at home in the country and within the diabetes and stem cell research communities that have embraced her work. "This is a great place to be scientist, to be a female scientist," she says, noting the incredible number of role models there are in this current generation of researchers. She is proud of the young scientists she is nurturing in her lab, who have developed the same passion and interest in diabetes she has—not just as cells in a dish—but as a condition that impacts the lives of real people. "They are dedicated to the lab, to the work, but they also want to find a cure."

There is also a spirit of collaboration in Canada that is not always possible in other research communities. Rather than competing, Nostro, Shapiro, Kieffer, MacDonald, and the many others in this research area are working together in an effort to move things forward faster.

Nostro sees so much more to come in this country where Till and McCulloch discovered the stem cells that fascinate her and where Banting, Best, Collip, and Macleod discovered insulin. "The scientists here are not just living off that legacy," she says. "They're shaping the field in type 2 diabetes and type 1 diabetes. It's exciting to be here at the crossroads of that."

She also has no doubt that, though it may take years to get there, the work being done in stem cells is going to one day have an impact on people living with diabetes. "It's not a question of *if* for me. It's a question of *when* this is going to happen."

CHAPTER SIX

It's All About the Beta Cells, Baby

When Dr. Jenny Bruin arrived at Ottawa's Carleton University, the challenges of leading a brand-new research program were immediately clear. Bruin, who had spent the last six-and-a-half years working in Dr. Timothy Kieffer's stem-cell focused lab at the University of British Columbia, was used to having state-of-the-art facilities for her work in stem cell biology at her fingertips. Now she had areas in her new lab that looked like a 1970s kitchen and a tight budget to balance while transforming it. She was both shell-shocked and completely thrilled.

"That was really eye-opening for me, having come from this fully functioning, really productive lab where everything happens immediately—or yesterday," she says. "And that was the mindset when I arrived, that I wanted to get going on day one, and then I had to really step back and realize just how much groundwork there was to get the lab to the point where we could do the most basic experiments."

The fact that Bruin had ended up at Carleton at all was a bit of a mystery to some in the research community. Seen as one of the best young researchers in Canada's growing stem cell and islet biology community, when Bruin took her first position as a PI or principal investigator, most expected it would be at a leading institute in the field. But it made sense that she chose Ottawa, where she has a family support system to help her balance parenting young children with building a lab. However, since the Ottawa Hospital Research Institute, led by Dr. Duncan Stewart, has a world-leading stem cell research program and Carleton had—prior to Bruin's arrival—exactly zero stem cell researchers, her choice was surprising to many.

But for Bruin, it was an easy decision. She liked the balance Carleton offered in terms of allowing her to teach while still focusing on research. While there were bigger research centres that were interested in having her, she felt that Carleton, with its recent push to expand its health sciences research program and their excitement about her work, would be a better fit.

"I really enjoy getting to know the students and influencing their path," she says. "I have a lot of undergrads in my lab who are trying to figure out if they like science, whether they want to go into research or medical school, and I feel like we have a real opportunity to influence their direction, both by teaching and exposing them early to research, so I like the balance where it's not all about research all the time. I feel like I'm a better researcher because of the teaching I do."

Bruin also realized that, despite the work she had already done and the reputation she had earned in stem cell science, it might be harder to carve out her own identity as an independent researcher in some of the bigger institutes. At Carleton, students seek her out and are eager to work in her lab. And because she is not relying solely on graduate students and postdoctoral fellows, she has the ability to be a mentor to undergrads who are just starting out in choosing a career path.

Dr. Bruce McKay, the director of the Institute of Biochemistry and an associate professor at Carleton, was part of the hiring committee who considered Bruin's application. Upon seeing her curriculum vitae, the extensive list of projects and publications expected of research scientists, Bruin was quickly short-listed and invited for an interview via Skype. McKay recalls that Bruin, who was eight months pregnant during her first interview, brought along her then two-month-old for the follow-up, with the infant making an adorably memorable impression on all.

McKay also liked that Bruin was able to provide medically relevant education, as well as cell culture and stem cell training to the students. He was impressed by her ability to bring in the very competitive funding grants needed to grow her lab, as well. Most importantly, he has since seen how much the students enjoy learning from her. "She's very energetic, and she's excited about her work, and that gets translated in part to the students who work with her."

Bruin's PhD student, Myriam Hoyeck, can attest to this. Hoyeck was considering her options for a Master's program when Bruin approached her. Bruin had noticed Hoyeck's impressive lab skills and asked the student to consider doing her Master's in Bruin's lab. Unfamiliar with her new professor's research background but inspired by her teaching skills, Hoyeck took a chance. She ended up loving the experience so much that she is now pursuing her PhD in Bruin's lab.

"I'm so glad she picked Carleton," says Hoyeck, noting that the type of health research Bruin does was not previously available at the school. Now it has opened up opportunities for students like herself to expand their options.

Hoyeck has learned much in the lab from Bruin, who gave her a solid foundation for basic research, but more than that, Bruin imparted on her the importance of treating everyone in the lab with the same level of respect. "One of the things I love about Jenny is that even though she is a PI, she never looks down on her students. Sometimes when people are really well-known in their field or they have a lot of knowledge, when you talk to them, you feel a bit belittled. It's not at all like that with Jenny," she says. "Everyone in the lab is equal. It doesn't matter if it's the PI, a grad student, or an undergrad, so I try to do that when I train students. I want to have that same relationship with everyone because it really helps the lab grow, and you feel comfortable asking questions."

While Hoyeck had never considered lab work focused on diabetes before her time with Bruin, now she hopes that helping those with this chronic disease will become a part of her career. "I would love to keep doing research in diabetes," she says. "There are so many potential questions that we can still answer."

* * * * *

Just a few years after moving to Carleton, Bruin is already in a space that is far removed from the 1970s kitchen she first found herself in. When I visit her in 2018, her lab is big and spacious and fully set up to do the complex work she thrives on. It is also poised for a move to a more suitable space for stem cell work in the building. She happily points out the large boxes lining the halls of the Biology Department that will soon be making their way into her revamped lab.

Bruin fits in at Carleton, where she has started a science communications course to help students better translate their work, and where she can concentrate on her current area of study, which focuses on environmental impacts on beta cells, the ones which produce insulin in our pancreas.

Science is in Bruin's blood. Her father was a science teacher—*her* chemistry teacher in high school, in fact, and many of her earliest memories are of doing science projects. "I was the only kindergarten student with an experiment at the science fair," she says with a laugh, recalling that the project involved combining colours to make new ones. "I had a Bristol board display with all of my findings. It's really funny when I look back on it, but I was so proud of it, and I got a ribbon."

The only one of her siblings to go into science, Bruin says her father didn't exert much pressure on his kids to get involved in research, but he definitely encouraged her work. To this day, he still reads all the new papers she publishes.

Now those papers are focused on the question of whether or not pollutants in our environment impact our beta cells even before we're born. With the rising rates of diabetes around the world, Bruin wondered what exactly was happening with our beta cells. "As a researcher, that fascinates me. We know that there's a genetic component to both type 1 and type 2 diabetes, but it doesn't explain the growing number of people with the disease," she says. "My lab is trying to understand which environmental factors might be influencing diabetes risk. And we're particularly interested in the beta cell. And once those cells are damaged, they can't really regenerate.

"Basically, the number of beta cells we're born with can set us up for life," she says. "So, if we're born with fewer beta cells, we're at a lifelong risk for developing diabetes." Then she started to wonder if perhaps the chemicals around us were responsible for beta cell death or dysfunction.

Bruin has focused on persistent pollutants—the ones that stick around for decades and can cause harm long after they might have originally been used. "There was one particular class of chemicals that jumped out to me as being consistently linked with an increased diabetes risk. And that was a class called dioxins or dioxin-like chemicals.

"We don't know from the human literature if exposure to these chemicals is causing diabetes. My lab is looking at whether exposure to this class of dioxin-like chemicals might be potentially causing beta cell death in adults. It's also possible that this exposure is occurring early or during pregnancy. For example, during pancreas development. It could be responsible for any adverse effects on pancreas development."

It's an interesting area of study, with lots of potential twists and turns for a researcher who has been credited with having developed some of the best stem-cell-derived beta cells in the world. This is high praise coming from the man who says it to me, Dr. Jim Johnson, a professor and researcher at the University of British Columbia. Johnson worked alongside Bruin while she was in Kieffer's lab, which shares space in the department with his own lab. An expert on beta cells, Johnson has been skeptical about those he's seen developed via stem cells in labs thus far, but he felt the ones that Bruin worked on alongside collaborator Dr. Alireza Rezania were on the right track.

"Jenny is an up-and-coming research star in the stem cell field. Her work established one of the leading protocols for taking pluripotent stem cells and turning them into cells that resemble pancreatic beta cells quite a bit," Johnson says. "The cells that Jenny was a part of making and studying were some of the closest I've seen yet."

Johnson's trajectory in researching beta cells is, in many ways, the opposite of Bruin's story. Though both started out in Ontario and ended up working at side-by-side labs in British Columbia, they are very different types of people. Bruin meets me at her lab in jeans and a sweater. Her brown hair is short and practical; her vibe is relaxed and serene. Johnson tends toward snappy suits paired with unique shirts. He zips around Vancouver in a fancy sports car, while Bruin drops me at the Ottawa airport in her practical four-door sedan. Johnson has a reputation for his willingness to fight for ideas that may buck the norms, while Bruin tends to emit a warm and nurturing energy.

Perhaps the greatest example of their differences is showcased in their arrivals at the Diabetes Canada offices to record their respective interviews with me for the podcast. Bruin pops into the office, and lets reception know she is there. She's chatty, relaxed, and happy to talk about her work as we head to the office where we will record. The next morning, I am scheduled to meet Johnson for our interview at 8:30 a.m. I get a text at 8:15 a.m. to say that he has arrived early, and I hurry to the office, not wanting to leave him sitting in the lobby. I shouldn't have worried. When I walk in, Johnson is holding court with the CEO and a cadre of staff who have been drawn in by the animated scientist. Wearing a designer shirt with a fascinating animal print, Johnson is chatting away about this research and is very much the life of this early-morning party.

Even their paths to science differ greatly. Bruin knew from kindergarten that science was in her blood. Johnson pursued numerous paths before settling on research. When he tells me his first plan was to study fine arts, this surprises me, as it's hard to picture the hockey-obsessed Johnson in a studio with a paintbrush. Instead, he detoured to studying kinesiology at Lakehead University in Thunder Bay, which also fed his love of sports.

At the end of his undergraduate degree, he decided to apply for graduate studies, and he readily admits that the partying and general slacking off he'd done in Thunder Bay meant he had limited success with landing a graduate position. Finally, one of his mentors, who felt Johnson had a lot of untapped potential, recommended him to Dr. John Chang in Edmonton. Chang ended up accepting him into his lab in the biological sciences department of the University of Alberta. There, Johnson finally found a role that fit, and he invested the energy he'd previously spent partying into learning everything he could about physiology.

Bruin fits right in at Carleton. Despite being in the heart of Canada's capital, it has a very small-town vibe, which suits her. However, I can't help but think that Johnson wouldn't find the same appeal. It's an interesting juxtaposition to talk to both researchers. They are both highly regarded in the field of beta cell biology and driven to find a way to end the type 2 diabetes epidemic. They are also interested in seeing all of the places where their work intersects and where it divides.

Johnson has one of those fancy state-of-the-art labs with a beautiful view of Vancouver—right next door to the one Bruin left behind. It's where he has spent more than fifteen years studying beta cell survival and function and how that affects diabetes.

Beta cells are at the heart of the pathology for all major types of diabetes. For those with type 1 diabetes, their beta cells have mostly been killed off by the immune system, though in recent years, there is research to suggest that there are still *some* functional beta cells.

In type 2 diabetes, there is beta cell dysfunction. This is an area Johnson is particularly interested in. What happens to our beta cells when type 2 diabetes develops? How can we protect them from stress? What can researchers discover in the lab that will help clinicians intervene in a meaningful way?

"Currently, all the treatments we have for diabetes treat the symptoms of the disease. They lower blood sugar," he explains. "There's nothing we have yet that can correct the fundamental problems with the beta cells. Our work in the lab is trying to identify and fix those underlying problems."

Johnson's research has shown enough promise that he has been able to work around the world. He did his postdoctoral studies in St. Louis with some of the top diabetes researchers in the U.S.—including Dr. Ken Polonsky and Dr. Stan Misler.

In 2004, Johnson landed his position at the University of British Columbia, and then he took a sabbatical to study at Oxford with one of the world's leading genetics teams in order to learn more about the genetics of diabetes. He then returned to Oxford when he was invited by Novo Nordisk to set up their type 2 diabetes research institute. He loves his work at UBC, but as we chat over tea in a café on Vancouver's Granville Island, he admits that he sometimes misses the unique research environment at Oxford.

Johnson seems indefatigable in his research interests. He attends more conferences than almost any researcher I know, whether to speak or just to learn, and he has an insatiable thirst for knowledge. While Bruin seems content to do excellent work in a lab full of students, Johnson seems to attack his research with the brute force and determination he uses as part of his regular hockey league games.

This is a quality that attracts students and post-docs who want to push the envelope a little bit. Dr. Gareth Lim did his postdoctoral studies in Johnson's lab before he moved into his current role as a Principal Investigator at Centre de recherche du CHUM in Montréal. Lim had previously trained in the lab of Toronto's Dr. Patricia Brubaker, one of Canada's most respected basic scientists.

Brubaker is at the forefront of GLP-1 and GLP-2 research in the world and was a key member of the research team that discovered a treatment for short bowel syndrome. Having spent time in her lab, Lim had a research background that was second to none, and Johnson's lab seemed like the right fit to take a deeper dive into the science he hoped to eventually do as a principal investigator. "I wanted to switch fields from my PhD training in the gut to pancreatic beta cell biology," he says. "For this work, it was important to be in an environment and research group that used multiple techniques and performed highly innovative experiments."

In Johnson's lab, well-reasoned creativity is encouraged, and Lim thrived. "Being able to embark on risky experiments and drive my own research projects were the best experiences," Lim says. "Jim gave me quite a bit of leeway to design and execute my projects. This degree of independence was critical for my training."

This willingness to take chances is something Lim sees as fundamental to Johnson's success as a scientist. "He challenges current dogmas and is not afraid to do so. Like all fields, there are dogmas and paradigms that have been unchallenged for a long time, and Jim has never been one to shy away from taking risks to challenge them."

Johnson's latest risk involves wading into the complicated world of diabetes and diet. He recently helped to found the Institute for Personalized Therapeutic Nutrition, a not-for-profit organization which aims to help health care providers and patients better understand personalized nutrition interventions. The idea that what someone eats can impact them on a metabolic level is incredibly interesting to Johnson. He wants to better understand why one person who eats a low-carbohydrate diet can put their type 2 diabetes into remission, while for another person, the diet has a negative effect.

What is going on in our cells that causes this to happen?

The work is controversial. For years, there has been a debate in the diabetes community about which diet is best—and for many, especially those in the type 1 diabetes community, the idea that any one diet can "cure" diabetes is frustrating and insulting. For those with type 2 diabetes, there is much more promise in this area of study, though it is still fraught with complexities and considerations.

Yet the research in this area fascinates Johnson, and the results from recent clinical trials, including one led by Dr. Jon Little at the University of British Columbia's Okanagan campus, provide hope that some patients with type 2 diabetes can stop taking their medications if they are able to stick to specific diets.

In the type 2 diabetes remission space, Johnson cites the basic science work of Dr. Marc Prentki—a professor of nutrition at the Université de Montréal—as a particular influence.

Prentki introduced the term *glucolipotoxicity*, which is a process involving nutrient excess that harms the beta cell and other tissues. He is looking at how the nutrients we eat move through our bodies and how they are detoxified along the way. How efficiently our bodies process nutrients could potentially have an impact on many things— like obesity or beta cell stress.

He is also leading research in the area of personalized nutrition— the idea that if we understand how our individual body metabolizes nutrients, we can eat a diet that is appropriate for us. For example, your friend who has been telling you he was able to stop his type 2 diabetes medications when he went vegan is right. However, if *you* go vegan, you may not experience the same results. Prentki and Johnson want to understand the metabolic reasons for this, which will ultimately help patients choose what diet is best suited for their own bodies.

Prentki likens this to the way we determine who should be on what medications. "Research in diabetes, obesity and cardiology shows that a given drug like insulin is good in some individuals and may be bad in others. Also, all too often, from the positive effects in a specific population of patients, it is concluded that a given drug is safe for all patients when this may not be the case."

It's a similar situation with nutrition, he explains, where not everyone following a specific diet will have a positive result, and yet we give people the same advice or suggest everyone eat similar diets. "You would expect that if you eat a lot of bread, your blood glucose level would necessarily go really high. And if you eat a lot of proteins or fibres, it would go low. This is true for a large fraction of people but not all. Some will have hyperglycemia eating proteins but not bread. The implication is that there is not a single optimal diet for all and that the future of personalized medicine should include personalized nutrition as well."

For Prentki, determining each person's specific phenotype and understanding how their body processes nutrients would help in determining the right diet for an individual. Johnson thinks this theory has merit, and through his role at the Institute for Personalized Nutrition, he hopes to further this type of study.

He's aware, though, that this work rankles many. In particular, those researchers who point out that while personalized nutrition is an incredible idea, in practice, it would be expensive, difficult to administer, and available only to those at a certain level of privilege. With type 2 diabetes being more prevalent in those of lower socioeconomic status and in marginalized and minority communities, is it a realistic goal to work toward?

"For me, there's two pieces. One piece is understanding human metabolic physiology, and that is different probably for different groups of people," Johnson says. However, he understands that this is a much more layered issue involving the second part—food insecurity, poverty, and the other inequalities that make focusing on just the physiological impossible. "Although I'm not an academic expert in the other aspect, you can't have one without the other."

Johnson knows this work is nuanced and will involve much more research. Ideally, he'd like to see diet studied in the same way we study the drugs that make their way to market. He uses current cardiovascular trials as an example. In order for a drug to be approved, there must be a five-year study involving thousands of participants. The trials cost millions of dollars and are most often funded by the pharmaceutical companies who want to bring their drug to market. "But what you end up with is a pretty accurate answer about what the drug does."

Having those answers about nutrients would allow for better research and could inform policy. A possibility? Maybe. But a long way off, if so. However, these types of long-term goals with potentially enormous payoffs drive Johnson. When we discuss the current work being done to build beta cells in the lab, he expresses doubt that one specific beta cell type could solve the problem of diabetes.

His lab has recently been interested in work showing that there are potentially different types of beta cells in the body. It's a novel idea, but one he finds intriguing. Johnson would love to see a bespoke beta cell production option in the future, developed expressly to work with the physiology of the individual person. It sounds like science fiction, and yet when you talk to him, it's hard not to think, "Why not?"

It is this desire to do the work that moves these ideas forward— whether they are ten or twenty or a hundred years in the future— that makes Johnson so interesting. One of his many ideas, coupled with his willingness to push the envelope, could be what leads to a major breakthrough. There is certainly enough talent and passion in his lab to produce it, or it may be that his team lays the groundwork for the next generation—the future Jim Johnsons—to take things even further.

The beta cell has captured the interest of thousands of researchers around the world. They want to know why it works, what happens when it doesn't, why it gets stressed, and how we could repair it. Bruin's quiet, methodical work in Ottawa may uncover some of those answers. Or it could instead be Johnson's bold ambitions that solve these problems. Both have already contributed much to assembling the puzzle.

Regardless, they are both inspiring and engaging a new generation of scientists, who are drawn to their unique personalities. Even just a few years into her first PI position, Bruin has already had an enormous influence on at least one student's future.

"I want to be her when I grow up," Myriam Hoyeck tells me. She is laughing as she says it, but as the undergrad who had never heard of Dr. Jenny Bruin's research before joining her lab has just received a 2020 CIHR Canadian Graduate Scholarship Award to pursue her PhD (she placed seventh out of 418 applicants), I suspect she's not entirely joking.

Neurons in the Pancreas

Dr. Derek van der Kooy is sitting a few rows ahead of me at an event featuring several student presentations, but he has leaned his head back and seems to be completely asleep. It's hard to blame him. While scientific presentations can be incredibly interesting, spending an hour in a stuffy room listening to young scientists shakily present their beginner findings is not exactly the most scintillating way to pass the time.

I'm not even paying that much attention myself, wondering instead at van der Kooy's ability to hold on to his iced coffee while asleep. Then, as the presentation ends and the moderator calls for questions, van der Kooy's head snaps up, and he raises his hand—asking a question so laser-focused that it proves he was clearly wide awake the whole time, listening to every word.

Van der Kooy is one of the most interesting characters in the Canadian research landscape. A talented and highly respected scientist whose work on stem cells in the brain has been recognized internationally, he is also a bit of a maverick. While most scientists rely on intricate PowerPoint slides rife with graphs and statistics to present their findings, van der Kooy tends to talk off the top of his head. It can be mesmerizing since he is able to make his point and share his science in a way that is both understandable to the average person and impressive to the scientific community. And he typically makes these presentations in his uniform of sorts—Bermuda shorts and baggy T-shirts. His grey hair pops up in unruly tufts as if there are simply far too many other important matters he has to attend to than brushing them back into place. It gives him a slight mad-scientist vibe.

Despite his quirks, or perhaps because of them, van der Kooy is beloved by many in the community and popular with students. Here too, he shows a certain flair. While he has many, shall we say, *traditional* graduate and postdoctoral students in his lab, he has also generated a reputation for encouraging and employing students who bring with them a more unique set of skills. Dr. Samantha Yammine is one of Canada's top science communicators, harnessing the power of social media to develop her "Science Sam" brand, all while successfully finishing her PhD under van der Kooy's watch.

Dr. Tahani Baakdhah is a well-known science artist who creates anatomically accurate crochet versions of cells and has even released a book of her patterns. She is a PhD student in van der Kooy's lab as well. He tells me that he once even had a Master's student who wanted to study the ethics of using neural stem cells in mice as part of his philosophy degree. Why not? van der Kooy thought, noting that the student, Dr. Phil Karpowitz, is now a successful scientist in his own right—and an associate professor at the University of Windsor.

So why is van der Kooy, who is arguably not a diabetes researcher, in this book? Well, as it happens, as part of his work studying the neurons of the brain, his lab made a discovery that might one day inform how beta cells are regenerated in the pancreas. Their discovery? That while about 85 percent of the neurons in the gut that cause food to move through our stomach and intestines are developed in the neuronal crest of the brain, the other 15 percent of those neurons of the gut are developed in—of all places—our pancreas.

This discovery was strange. So strange, in fact, that when his students first showed him the results of their work, van der Kooy made sure they checked multiple times that they hadn't accidentally contaminated their cultures with the neurons they regularly work with in his lab. But, no, it turns out that they were there. And they were on the move. The neurons, they found, migrated from the pancreas to the local nervous system that surrounds the intestine. "We suggested that neurons produced by pancreatic stem cells are an evolutionary leftover," he says. "The pancreas first evolved in an early multicellular ancestor by expressing a neuronal program in a gut cell."

This has many implications in terms of the evolutionary history of our pancreas, but for van der Kooy, the fact that this organ made neurons and that they were connected to the gut was interesting. Could that mean that a pancreatic beta cell could actually be convinced to reproduce in the pancreas itself? "The rare pancreatic stem cells make a few neurons, but they also make all of the cells of the pancreas, including the insulin-producing beta cells." Thus, it wasn't so much the neurons produced by the pancreas that struck the team, but the discovery that beta cells were produced by the pancreatic stem cells. This suggested that endogenous adult pancreatic stem cells might be able to produce new beta cells to treat people living with diabetes.

Scientists around the world are currently trying to figure out how to create beta cells in the lab and how to keep them alive once they are implanted. This could, in theory, cure type 1 diabetes. But as van der Kooy's team studied the pancreas, their discovery of these neurons opened up another idea for him. "The discovery of endogenous pancreatic stem cells provides another way of thinking about it. Can we actually get pancreatic stem cells to make new insulin-producing beta cells *in vivo*?"

Through experiments, his lab has shown that the stem cells of a mouse or a person with diabetes are *always* trying to make new cells. Stem cells from those with diabetes, surprisingly, proliferate more than those without. He thinks this occurs because the cells try to replace the ones that are missing. But because the body continues to attack the cells, they don't survive.

Of course, if someone could develop new cells in their body, what can be done to keep the immune system from destroying those new cells in the same way it destroyed the original cells and caused type 1 diabetes in the first place? Van der Kooy gets visibly excited discussing this—he lives with type 1, which gives him an extra layer of interest in the topic.

Perhaps, van der Kooy posits, it's not about replacing the ones that have been lost, but in stopping the autoimmune attack in the first place. He's currently working on a project with Dr. Andras Nagy, funded by Toronto's Medicine by Design, that is looking at just that.

"Can we find a neat way to protect the cells immunologically? And if we can, is there a way to actually, endogenously, with drugs that stimulate the pancreatic stem cells, to make new beta cells that would replace the ones in diabetes?"

As he talks, it's hard not to get caught up in the wonder of all this. Could the body of someone with type 1 diabetes simply regenerate new beta cells and develop new islets, if their immune system was reprogrammed not to attack the cells?

Sitting in his office at the University of Toronto, listening to van der Kooy explain all this at breakneck speed, completely enraptured by the potential of these cells, I feel like I'm getting a sneak peek inside the way his brain untangles these biological mysteries. Understanding the evolution of our biology—how our body develops from a tiny embryo into all the pieces that make up who we are—brings us tiny steps closer to being able to fix the things inside us that break.

Could it be that a few busy neurons that grew in our pancreas hold the key? Maybe. And if so, will van der Kooy wear a T-shirt when he accepts all the awards this discovery might bring? Likely.

CHAPTER SEVEN

Creating the Cycle

Dr. Rémi Rabasa-Lhoret rode his bicycle to work on a snowy day in Montréal just before he sat down with me for an interview. He jokes about this later on, as he shares his hope that the weather in Toronto, where I'm calling him from, is better. On its face, this is not unusual, but I can't help wondering if the leadership teams at the Université de Montréal—where he is a professor—and the Montréal Clinical Research Institute—where he is vice president of clinic and clinical research—would like one of their research superstars risking life and limb on Montréal's treacherous winter roads.

Born and raised in France, Rabasa-Lhoret did not anticipate spending his career in Québec, yet it's in this province where he's built a reputation as one of the premier diabetes researchers in the country—if not the world. We are talking today about his work on the artificial pancreas, a project that has consumed much of his time for more than ten years and which has the potential to have an enormous impact on those living with type 1 diabetes.

With the advent of insulin pumps, continuous glucose monitors, and other forms of technology to ease the burden of diabetes management, there has long been discussion of the possibility of an artificial pancreas. In the 1970s, Dr. Bernard Leibel and Dr. Michael Albisser from Mount Sinai Hospital in Toronto built an early prototype—it showed that the ability to manage insulin delivery in an automated fashion was possible, but it was extremely large and cumbersome, nothing like today's devices.

While the new technologies help to automate the process of monitoring and managing blood sugars, in some ways they also increase the complexity. The device allows people to better understand and control the fluctuations they experience, which in turn reduces the risk of complications, but the process is far from intuitive and certainly not automated—and the artificial pancreas would change that.

Rabasa-Lhoret's lab is not the only one working on this project, as many teams around the world are also hard at work trying to develop a piece of wearable tech that would transform diabetes management. Yet Rabasa-Lhoret and his collaborator, Dr. Ahmad Haidar from McGill University, have developed one of the most promising options. Their version, a dual-hormone artificial pancreas, aims to automate the use of both insulin and other add-on drugs, such as glucagon, for the patient, allowing them to go about their life never having to worry about their blood sugar skyrocketing too high or dipping too low.

"The artificial pancreas was always a long-term desire," Rabasa-Lhoret explains. "When I was training in France in 1999, I was able to see the first attempt for an implanted pump with an implanted sensor and complete closed loop just before I left. It was fascinating to see that we were close enough to test this on a patient."

The concept stuck with him and became a focus of his research after he moved to Canada permanently in 2002. However, it wasn't until around 2010, when he received an application from Haidar, then a young engineer, that he felt he had found the missing piece of the puzzle needed to develop a prototype that could work.

"I had some ideas; he had some other ideas and the technical knowledge, we shared the passion," says Rabasa-Lhoret. "We were lucky that in the first study we had some good indication that we were going in the right direction. Though very far from a commercial product, we would be able to reduce hypoglycemia, to do this safer, to do this better, and were already envisioning that we could automate everything, or most of it, by making it simpler."

For Haidar's part, the connection to Rabasa-Lhoret helped him move forward a project that had started calling to him during his PhD studies. Originally from Lebanon, he had done his engineering training at the Kuwait University before deciding to pursue a Master's and PhD in Québec—this despite the fact that he spoke no French at all. During a visit back to his alma mater, he was invited to attend some student talks. "Me, being a big geek, on my holidays, I decided to go and attend these presentations," he says with a chuckle. "One of them was on control systems for diabetes in engineering, and that grabbed my attention."

Haidar had been looking for a medical application to better develop his engineering expertise, and the presentation he saw sparked the idea that a closed-loop system for an artificial pancreas—one where both monitoring glucose levels and insulin injections were automated—was the perfect opportunity. Sensors to track glucose levels had recently become available on the market, making it possible for someone with diabetes to track their blood sugar levels more easily and making the idea of an automated system to manage insulin administration much more realistic.

Returning to Montréal, Haidar read all he could about the process and approached his supervisor with the idea of working on an artificial pancreas. His supervisor suggested he talk to Dr. Laurent Legault, then the head of the insulin pump centre at Montréal Children's Hospital. Legault was excited about the potential of what Haidar wanted to do. However, he did not have access to the facilities needed to support a clinical research project of that scope, which would involve patients spending 24 to 48 hours in the hospital to have their glucose levels closely monitored—a timeframe that was necessary to effectively test the type of system Haidar wanted to build.

"When Ahmad came to meet me with the idea, I saw that he was well-read in the field of diabetes and was eager to include children in his research endeavours, which obviously got my attention," Legault says. "Skilled engineers frequently lack the clinical training to understand how their technology could impact actual patients. It was clear, after my long discussion with Ahmad, that this not only had potential but was also doable."

Legault suggested Haidar contact a colleague, Dr. Rémi Rabasa-Lhoret, whose position at the Montréal Clinical Research Institute gave him access to the resources for such an endeavour, and who also had a deep interest in this type of project.

And thus a collaboration was born, with all three men heavily invested in the idea that they could create something that would make life easier for someone living with diabetes. Haidar took a year to study in Cambridge under one of the leading experts in the area of closed-loop technology. At the same time, he applied with Rabasa-Lhoret and Legault for the funding they would need to start a project in Québec. In 2011, when he returned to Canada flush with knowledge, the team received small grants from Diabetes Canada and Diabetes Québec that allowed them to start work on their idea.

From the outset, this project had a momentum rare in health care research. All three collaborators felt they were onto something. Working in Canada presented challenges—they had far fewer resources than the labs at Cambridge and Harvard that were also working on prototypes—but in other ways it was helpful, as it forced them to be creative. Their funders were very supportive of the work, and the Québec team was the only one in the country working on this type of technology, which meant less competition for the money they needed.

"We could be in a position to help hundreds of children achieve better control and improve safety with the help of currently used technologies," recalls Legault. "Montréal Children's Hospital was at the forefront of the diabetes technology movement, creating the first freestanding insulin pump centre in the province. The pump *is* a powerful tool, but most families did not use it to its full potential. Glucose monitors were also starting to be used, but it was somewhat difficult to figure how to best use them." The artificial pancreas, he felt, would create a more seamless technology.

While other labs might be rushing to get a prototype to market, Rabasa-Lhoret and Haidar turned their attention to rigorous science. They published fewer papers, but those that they did were considered among the strongest worldwide and helped pave the way for the first generation of closed-loop technologies that started to hit the market in 2018.

These first-generation devices are a big step forward, but they are insulin only. So that means that while they help to automate the process of people living with type 1 diabetes by monitoring sugar levels and administering glucose as needed, there is still a level of management that rests with the person using the device.

For Rabasa-Lhoret and Haidar, the dream is to find a way to automate the entire process. "The ultimate goal is really the fully closed-loop system, where you wear the system, you eat, and you don't need to think about delivering insulin at mealtime," says Haidar. "You just eat what you want, and you feel free in your dietary choices."

Rabasa-Lhoret sees the current insulin-only, closed-loop systems as great progress, but he knows that for patients, they are not enough. "The analogy I would use is that you drive your diabetes. If it was a car, you're just lying on the accelerator. You just push more or less and sometimes even take your foot off the accelerator for a bit, like when you drive on the highway, and there's not too much traffic," he explains. The dual-hormone version he hopes for is more nuanced. With an insulin-only device, someone who goes extremely low would still need to either take rapid-absorbing sugar or administer glucagon to treat this. The dual-hormone pump, on the other hand, would register the need and provide glucagon automatically, just like when you push the brakes on your car to avoid an accident.

Legault credits Haidar with presenting him with the initial idea of a dual hormone artificial pancreas, understanding that both insulin and glucagon are missing in those with type 1 diabetes. "Glucagon was meant to prevent hypoglycemia in situations where the risk for it increases, like during exercise or between meals," he says. "In pediatrics, we use glucagon in mini doses to rescue patients from an emergency visit, and that concept was embedded in the design of the artificial pancreas. Our results clearly showed that we were improving glucose levels without increasing hypoglycemia. While not perfect, and not a cure, this approach is available now and could lead to a dramatic improvement in care."

I have always found it interesting that so few of the diabetes researchers I have met have a personal connection to diabetes when they begin their work. Yet as they continue in the field, their dedication to those living with the disease becomes deeply etched into their projects. Rabasa-Lhoret had never considered studying diabetes until his residency in France when his supervisor encouraged him to work on a project dealing with type 1 diabetes. It stirred an interest that never waned.

Similarly, Haidar admits that his decision to work in diabetes was purely one of professional interest at the time. He had seen a use for his engineering skills to solve a medical need, and he decided to pursue it. As his work brought him deeper into the diabetes community, his general interest turned into a calling.

For both men, the opportunity to do their research at a camp for children with type 1 diabetes created an even stronger bond to the community. Situated along the shores of Lac Didi, near Sainte-Agathe-des-Monts in Québec's Laurentians, Camp Carowanis is a summer camp specially designed to give children and youth with type 1 diabetes a traditional camp experience, with the medical supervision needed to ensure a safe, exciting week or two away from home. It was there that Rabasa-Lhoret and Haidar spent two summers, experiencing firsthand the lives of young people living with diabetes and doing the type of research that may one day transform the lives of those with the disease.

Working in a camp setting, Haidar explains, is an incredible opportunity. The first year they went to Camp Carowanis, in 2014, they had more than thirty campers enrolled in a study that monitored and controlled their blood glucose levels overnight. When they returned in 2018, they had more than seventy. To get that number of patients involved in a hospital study could take two years, but at a camp where everyone has type 1 diabetes, and everyone is invested in finding new technologies to improve care, it becomes much easier to support this type of project.

Rabasa-Lhoret notes with a chuckle that he and Haidar were seen as very cool at camp—because everyone wanted to be involved in the study. "It's a lot of work, but then you get your study and your data accumulated in a supersonic way," he says, noting that it can be very hard to recruit people for studies when patients are managing school and work. When everyone is at camp already, and the project is built into the camp experience, it's much easier.

The time at camp allowed the research team to monitor blood sugar levels in a continuous way—during sleep and after meals—to help test the algorithms for their closed-loop device. While access to patients in this setting is helpful, it is also not an entirely natural environment. The camp is medically supervised to ensure everyone is safe, but it also takes people out of their typical day-to-day lives. There is much more physical activity and play, which increases the risk of overnight hypoglycemia. Meals may be different than what someone would normally eat, and factors like the weather can make planning unpredictable. It's not a perfect situation, but it's certainly better than most researchers can manage when looking to develop a system for an artificial pancreas.

It has also changed the way the two men work in diabetes. Rabasa-Lhoret was already a practicing clinician and very passionate about diabetes research when this opportunity arose but being around these young people had a profound impact on him. Haidar, who had come from an engineering background and had not worked directly with those with diabetes before, was even more affected.

"We love it at the camp. We are there 24 hours a day, but we aren't focused on our studies for all those 24 hours. In between, you interact with the kids, and you see what activity you can do to learn more about how people live with diabetes," he says. "After a while, you just feel like you are a part of that community. It's not about, 'I'm doing research on these kids and trying to publish,' it's more like this is my job as part of the type 1 diabetes community to do research and advance knowledge."

The information gathered during the camp studies has done much to further the team's work on the artificial pancreas. The algorithm Haidar developed has been adopted by a large pharmaceutical company for future use in their closed-loop system, and both researchers continue, separately, to study the use of glucagon and other add-on therapies for the next generation of closed loop. The focus and the rigour they are known for has drawn worldwide accolades, and their studies have helped move the field forward in terms of understanding the risks and rewards of using an automated system.

Haidar completed his PhD and postdoctoral studies and has since moved to a position at McGill, where he runs his own lab. There he is training the next generation of students and using the exceptional resources available to him—including a clinical investigation unit—to further refine the artificial pancreas. He is focused on developing algorithms that will help provide people with diabetes a fully automated experience, which includes exploring options beyond insulin and glucagon. He is also working closely with Dr. Bruce Perkins from Toronto to see if Perkins' work on SGLT2 inhibitors in type 1 diabetes could have practical applications in an artificial pancreas. Haidar's most recent version of an artificial pancreas is insulin-only, but as he tests and refines the process, the future holds much promise for a dual system.

Nancy Cardinez, a research nurse practitioner from Perkins' lab, plays a key role in the current clinical trials to test Haidar's artificial pancreas alongside the use of SGLT2 inhibitors. Approved for use in type 2 diabetes, these drugs remain unapproved for use outside clinical trials in type 1 diabetes in North America. This is due to the increased risk of diabetic ketoacidosis, a potentially life-threatening condition where the body produces excess ketones, which are a type of blood acids. However, many in the field believe there is enough promise from these drugs to warrant testing ways to include them in the treatment of type 1 diabetes. The Haidar/Perkins research project is one of the first of its kind internationally, and Cardinez has seen how eager patients are to participate in the trials.

"I think patients are very excited because they want to know about new research. They want to be involved with the new technological advances and novel diabetes management therapies. Most patients involved in our research are very keen on trying to improve their diabetes management and interested in various techniques to meet their glycemic targets," she says.

In her role, Cardinez is working closely with Haidar's team to ensure patients in the Toronto arm of the trial understand the complex technology and are able to troubleshoot any potential problems. She knows those who have agreed to be part of the trial are excited by the prospect of one day soon being able to manage their glucose in a more automated way—one that reduces the burden of carbohydrate counting and lessens the risk of hypoglycemia. However, Cardinez's role is to mitigate the risks they are taking on in being the first to try these new therapies that are not yet proven.

This is the first time Cardinez has worked with biomedical engineers, who are taking advanced engineering principles and trying to create technologies that will fit into the lives of patients. She is helping to bridge the gap and ensure the questions and concerns of patients are heard by the researchers and that the patient education materials developed are actually relevant for the end users. "It's very interesting to see the engineering side," she says. "That has been the biggest learning curve, to be involved in what goes into creating these systems and these studies, and how to now integrate the patient's side and the clinical perspective into that the process."

This blend of clinical and engineering work is at the heart of the artificial pancreas project in Canada.

"In engineering, we are wired to think about solutions. As part of our training, there is lots of emphasis on design. So when I go and see traces of sugar levels in someone with type 1 diabetes, the first thing that comes to my mind is how I can design something to change these," Haidar says.

"The reason you don't hear a lot about engineering is because engineers are typically working in industry, not in academia. The insulin pump was developed by engineers, and the glucose meter was developed by engineers. All these types of technology come from engineers, but typically they don't go sit at universities. Instead, they stay in industry and build new systems." Developing a research program that combines the patient, clinical, and engineering models drives Haidar's current work as he builds his team at McGill.

While Rabasa-Lhoret and Haidar no longer collaborate regularly, Rabasa-Lhoret continues to be involved in research on these technologies. Now, though, he spends a good deal of his time working on other projects, including his leadership role at IRCM and the BETTER Project, which looks at patient-focused ways to reduce hypoglycemia in type 1 diabetes.

Much of Rabasa-Lhoret's early interest in the artificial pancreas was in the role it could play in hypoglycemia prevention, which would substantially improve the lives of people living with diabetes, and that thread continues throughout all of his research projects. In addition, he is making an enormous contribution in a less well-known area of diabetes research—that of diabetes in those with cystic fibrosis (CF). Montréal and Toronto have two of the largest cystic fibrosis clinics in North America, and as a practicing endocrinologist, Rabasa-Lhoret has become aware of the unique issues faced by this patient group. As treatments for cystic fibrosis have improved, people live longer, but they are also at an increased risk of developing a form of diabetes.

Rabasa-Lhoret was intrigued when he saw that patients with CF who lived to be forty had an almost 80 percent chance of having some form of abnormal glucose. "It's not type 1, it's not type 2, but it has some parts of both," he explains. "There's a long prediabetes phase like in type 2, but most of them are quite young and lean like in type 1. And usually, they will need insulin, also like in type 1."

It turns out that typical methods of screening for diabetes are also more challenging with CF patients. The fasting blood sugar tests that are most commonly used are less reliable in this population, as are A1C tests. That means that someone with CF needs to do an older-model glucose solution test and provide blood samples over two hours. This is cumbersome and less than ideal for patients with a condition that makes exposure to germs and viruses dangerous. Rabasa-Lhoret is now looking at ways to simplify this testing process to decrease the time in a medical setting and to take advantage of advances in continuous glucose-monitoring technology.

Working with CF patients with diabetes has brought with it all sorts of new challenges and insights on which Rabasa-Lhoret thrives. His CF patients don't worry about the same diabetes complications as his type 1 patients. No one thinks about their eyes or their kidneys when they are so focused on their extreme lung disease. He has had to adjust his thinking in that regard. And the insulin-induced weight gain that his diabetes patients worry about? For those with CF, where weight gain is often much-needed, this potential side effect is looked at positively.

Rabasa-Lhoret has found the work challenging and exciting. There are very few other researchers focused in this area, and his lab is considered one of the best in the world. It has also allowed him to see real, tangible results. "Simplifying the screening and trying to dissect the connection between diabetes, low lung function, and lower weight has the potential to increase life expectancy."

For Haidar, his inspiration continues to come from the children he met over his two summers at Camp Carowanis. When I ask him what he's most proud of in his career, he talks about his students and his work but then goes right back to his camp experience.

"There is one project we did last year in the camp that I feel extremely proud of," he says. The campground, he notes, is quite large. When he was doing his study, it would take him about ninety minutes to go around to each tent to make sure all the systems were working, and the sugar levels of the campers were fine. As more of the kids started to wear glucose sensors—a common accessory for anyone with type 1 diabetes who can afford it these days—he thought there must be a way to better monitor their sugar levels since checking every ninety minutes seemed less than optimal.

A glucose sensor can alert you to a low, but only if you hear or see it. "If a kid is sleeping 500 metres away from you and they have a hypo, and you are in the infirmary, you wouldn't know about it. Knowing about it in the morning is not helpful," he says.

So Haidar built a system that would allow the staff to monitor each child's glucose remotely. Working with several of his students, he developed a technology that could read each child's sensor and send the results wirelessly in real time to a display monitor in the infirmary. Suddenly, the medical team had the ability to know immediately if a child was dealing with hypoglycemia.

"This is not something we're publishing in a scientific journal," Haidar says, noting that the typical measure of scientific success doesn't apply here, but the technology has already had an enormous impact. "When we presented this system to the camp staff, some of the nurses were crying because it was such a life changer," he says. "I feel more proud of this project than any of the others. I felt that I changed people's lives right away. It's not something you have to wait for five years to see the change. If we don't do work in artificial pancreas research, someone else will do it at some point, but this is a local camp, and if I didn't do it, no one would do it."

It seems like an unlikely scenario that a clinician-scientist from France and an engineer from Lebanon would meet in Québec and develop a research program together that will have a substantial impact on the diabetes landscape far into the future. Yet, for all their differences in background and expertise, the core desire to improve the lives and reduce the burden of those who live with diabetes is at the heart of their collaboration and continued success.

CHAPTER EIGHT

Ladies First

We are having a belated fortieth birthday celebration, scarfing down pasta and sipping sparkling wine when my friend Tara drops her bombshell. She has been diagnosed with prediabetes. She makes a joke about how she is eating all the wrong things, but I can see the stress in her eyes. The news that she has prediabetes seems completely surreal coming from Tara, who is blessed with beautiful curves. She is not at all an obvious candidate for diabetes this early in her life. However, she does have polycystic ovary syndrome (PCOS), which makes her more likely to develop type 2 diabetes than someone without the condition.

Diabetes is one of those diseases that likes to join its friends in our bodies. It often aligns with heart disease, cancer, and a lot of other things we dread. People with mental illnesses, such as depression or schizophrenia, are also much more likely to be diagnosed with diabetes. And for women, there is a unique set of circumstances that seem to bring on type 2 diabetes when they least expect it.

PCOS causes an overabundance of male hormones in a woman's body, which can wreak havoc on her menstrual cycles and increase insulin resistance, among other things. Women who live with PCOS are also much more likely to develop type 2 diabetes. An Australian study of 8,000 women with PCOS found they were between 4 and 8.8 times more likely than women without PCOS to develop the disease. The reasons for this are varied, including increased insulin sensitivity and a higher likelihood of obesity in women with the condition. This seems especially unfair because they are already dealing with PCOS, which is often accompanied by other health issues. Tara, a freelance writer and editor, has had endometriosis, a painful condition where uterine tissue grows outside the uterus, since her teens, and struggles with other issues related to her reproductive health.

That she may need to worry about type 2 diabetes is a blow. Tara is aware of the stigma that can accompany the disease, and as she explained to me that day at the restaurant, she also felt a crushing sense of anxiety that she was not going to be able to beat the odds. That no matter how hard she tried to adapt her diet and lifestyle, she was still going to end up going from prediabetes to diabetes, and that this would be another way her body had failed her. It was heartbreaking to hear her say that, especially knowing that no matter how much of an effort she makes, the genetic odds may just not be in her favour. And that is definitely *not* her fault.

"The diagnosis made me feel two things: validation and fear. I knew instinctively that something was off in my body and that I would have to advocate for myself to get it properly checked out. So I was happy that I was able to bypass my GP's conclusion that 'everything is fine' and finally get to the bottom of it," she says now. "Even though a part of me intellectually realized that having PCOS makes me predisposed to getting diabetes, I still felt like it was somehow my fault. That I didn't have the willpower to avoid chips or ice cream when I knew I was getting older, and my body might be heading in that direction."

Prediabetes is typically defined as blood sugar that is higher than normal but not yet high enough to be considered full-blown type 2 diabetes. It is a common diagnosis (Diabetes Canada estimates that roughly six million people in the country are living with it), and more than half of those who have it will go on to develop type 2 diabetes. In Tara's case, she does not have elevated blood sugar levels but instead suffers from incredible lows or hypoglycemia. This is far less common, and it made it more difficult for her to figure out what was at the root of her scary symptoms.

"In the months leading up to my diagnosis, I had begun experiencing a lot of sugar-crash symptoms and cravings," she says. "During these episodes, I would start sweating, and my hands would shake. I would feel frantic like I needed to ingest something sweet immediately. I would also become very irritable and somewhat disoriented."

Aware from her own research into the condition that PCOS made her more prone to developing diabetes, Tara went to her family doctor for routine blood tests—and her fasting blood sugar came back at 4.8, well below the threshold for diabetes. So, all was normal, according to her doctor. Only it wasn't. Frustrated with the lack of answers, Tara insisted on seeing an endocrinologist.

"She took my concerns seriously, given my PCOS history," Tara says. "She also told me I was insulin resistant and had prediabetes, but that I also had reactive hypoglycemia, which meant that when I ate a high-glycemic-index food or high-carb meal, my cells weren't responding to my insulin properly, so my pancreas was sending a flood of insulin to compensate. This, in turn, caused my blood sugar levels to crash at a rapid rate. When I started monitoring my glucose levels, they would sometimes go as low as 3.2 or 3.4."

Now she is working to manage blood sugar levels using a continuous glucose monitoring device that helps her automatically track any fluctuations. She is eating healthier and trying to be as active as possible despite her health issues, but it isn't easy.

Tara admits that though she knows the occasional treat—like the half a glass of sparkling wine and some pasta we had at her birthday celebration—is fine to indulge in now and then, she often feels guilty if she is not able to be live up to the perfection she thinks others expect. "I still feel a certain stigma. I've told my close friends and family about it, but I do sense a certain judgment from people sometimes if I fall off the wagon and have a glass of wine or indulge in some birthday cake. It's like I feel a pressure to be this clean-eating role model all the time, and I just can't do it, especially around certain times of the month, when my cravings for carbs become much stronger."

Tara's case isn't the typical diabetes story given the connection to PCOS, but it does highlight something clinicians and scientists have been speaking about much more frequently of late—the unique health concerns of women. For decades, medical research tended to focus only on men. In recent years, however, it has become clear that this tendency to look at disease treatments through a one-size-fits-all lens isn't working.

This desire to provide better treatments to women with diabetes is what fuels the work of Toronto's Dr. Lorraine Lipscombe. An endocrinologist and scientist at Toronto's Women's College Hospital, she has spent her career studying the unique health issues women face and looking for solutions that will meet their needs. In her work as an endocrinologist, she realized there were challenges her female patients faced that weren't being adequately addressed, and she wanted to change that.

Lipscombe knew, for example, that there was evidence showing that one risk factor for breast cancer—a primarily female diagnosis—was obesity. She was also aware that many people living with type 2 diabetes also struggled with increased weight. She had seen research showing that having diabetes in and of itself could be a risk factor for breast cancer, regardless of the person's weight.

"We think this is due to the excess insulin that women who have type 2 diabetes have to produce in order to overcome the insulin resistance that characterizes type 2 diabetes," she explains. "And why would that be a concern? Well, insulin itself, when it's produced in the body, in addition to helping lower your blood glucose, also acts as a growth factor. Studies have shown that insulin can promote the growth of tumours—and in some cases, can even promote the *development* of tumours."

Lipscombe and her team wanted to know if what they had hypothesized in the lab was actually happening in the real world. To do this, she needed to closely study the rates of breast cancer in women with type 2 diabetes, so she decided to do it through the available medical information from the province. "We used the Ontario Health Care Databases to look at that question, and sure enough, we found that women have a small but significant increase of developing breast cancer after getting diabetes."

The risk, which has since been confirmed by other studies around the world, is a small one—about 10 percent—but Lipscombe learned two important reasons why this area needed increased study. "We know that by improving lifestyle, lowering weight, and improving insulin resistance, that this reduces the risk of diabetes and the complications of diabetes. But does it also reduce the risk of breast cancer?

"We've also shown in our previous work that because women with diabetes have a lot of health care needs and appointments and things to discuss with their doctors, there's evidence that they may not be getting their mammograms as often as they should. That's something to be aware of, and the best thing we can do right now is to ensure that women with diabetes, like women without diabetes, get their mammograms regularly after menopause."

While it may seem counterintuitive that those women who go to the doctor *more* don't get all the tests they need, it's actually fairly common. When you have so many obvious things to think about, something hidden, like breast cancer, can fall to the bottom of the pile.

Lipscombe has also been looking at ways to prevent women from developing type 2 diabetes in the first place. For some, like my friend Tara, genetic factors or other underlying conditions will play a part, but for others, lifestyle changes can make a significant difference. One such instance of this is gestational diabetes.

Gestational diabetes is a uniquely female issue, and it has long been shrugged off by the general public as not a big deal because it typically goes away after pregnancy. However, a huge swath of research now exists showing that women who have gestational diabetes in pregnancy are much more likely to develop type 2 diabetes later in life. While Tara did not experience gestational diabetes during her pregnancy, if she had, it could have been a signal—like the canary in the coal mine—that something was amiss with her insulin resistance and beta cell function.

Toronto's Dr. Ravi Retnakaran, from the Lunenfeld-Tanenbaum Research Institute at Mount Sinai Hospital, is another researcher looking at the way gestational diabetes may act as a signal for future diabetes risk. "Pregnancy is the best test for beta cell function we have," he explains. "It's normal for a woman, in the latter half of pregnancy, to be extremely resistant to insulin. That's normal physiology that will happen to all women in pregnancy. But only *some* women are going to develop gestational diabetes. These are women whose beta cells aren't able to respond appropriately to this test."

Pregnancy, he notes, is the only situation in medicine where we screen an entire part of the population for diabetes. "It's the perfect confluence of the best physiologic test your body's ever going to see for a future risk of diabetes, coupled with the fact that we actually do clinical testing."

For Retnakaran, this gives him a chance to study the pancreatic beta cells of women with and without gestational diabetes, looking at how the cells have developed and how to change them over time. If he can figure out the physiology, he could perhaps figure out why some women have this defect and others don't— and potentially— how to fix it. This is a long-term project linked to Retnakaran's work with methods to reverse type 2 diabetes, and while it is incredibly promising, it doesn't do much to help the day-to-day lives of women who are living with gestational diabetes right now. This is where re-searchers like Lipscombe are key.

Lipscombe's health coaching program is designed specifically to meet the needs of women who developed gestational diabetes in pregnancy, looking at the realities of life with new babies and the challenges of making significant lifestyle modifications during this period. It aims to change the trajectory for women with gestational diabetes and reduce their risk for developing type 2 diabetes later in life. The program has gone through a successful pilot and is head-ing into a clinical trial at the time of our first interview, which takes place in Lipscombe's bright and spacious office in the spring of 2018. Her face lights up as she explains the project and how it truly takes the unique needs of women and mothers into consideration.

In a nutshell, when a woman is diagnosed with gestational diabe-tes, she can be referred to the program after giving birth. She is then paired with a health coach. Lipscombe has partnered with diabetes educators, who have extensive knowledge about the disease and also benefit from the additional training they receive by participating in the project. The diabetes educators then set up regular phone calls with the women to help support their lifestyle changes. The reality of having a new baby makes it extremely difficult to make it to in-person meetings, so the phone calls, which are only ten to fifteen minutes long, remove a barrier and ease stress while still providing needed accountability. For six months, the new mom has a health coach supporting her in realistic ways to incorporate healthy eating habits and exercise into a life with a new baby.

"We know that type 2 diabetes can be prevented or delayed with healthy behaviour changes and weight loss in high-risk individuals, but we have very little evidence for women who've had gestational diabetes. We know that if they make lifestyle changes when they're becoming older, that this will reduce their risk of developing type 2 diabetes. But we feel we need to be intervening at a lot younger age because our data shows that up to twenty percent of women will be diagnosed with type 2 diabetes within ten years of a pregnancy with gestational diabetes," she says.

"Our program is looking at how we can provide education and support for women to be able to make these effective, healthy behaviour changes in a very demanding period of their life when they're starting their families. They've just had a baby, so there's a lot of changes already going on in their life and in their body. How can we engage those women and help them? We know that they want to make changes, and they are motivated, but life is busy, and they're exhausted. So many people have tried to provide them with support and have not been successful. We've made a few changes and adopted a few strategies to enhance that support, to make sure that we're able to provide what they need during that particular period of time."

About thirty percent of the time, glucose intolerance persists after a woman with gestational diabetes gives birth. In those cases, the woman may actually have had undiagnosed type 2 diabetes or prediabetes before she got pregnant. "It's really important for women who've had this condition in pregnancy to have a diabetes test within the first six months of when they've delivered," explains Lipscombe. "Because if they do already have some glucose intolerance, that has implications for future pregnancy planning. We want to make sure they are able to optimize their blood sugar control in the planning stage *and* in the early stages when the baby's organs are developing during the next pregnancy. If the condition has resolved and they don't have residual glucose intolerance, we still recommend they make healthy lifestyle changes to try and reduce their risk of getting gestational diabetes in a subsequent pregnancy. That's part of what we're looking at in our study."

The reality, though, is that most women in Canada aren't getting the follow-up they need. And many who go on to develop gestational diabetes in pregnancy don't get a lot of support after they give birth.

For Carly Mladenovsky, who lives in Whitby, Ontario, a gestational diabetes diagnosis was the last thing she expected. An active and fit person who enjoys exercise, she'd loved being pregnant with her son, Charlie, and the first-time mom hadn't experienced any of the sickness or discomfort she had feared in pregnancy. When her results came in at 27 weeks, it brought up a host of fears. "I was shocked at first, and really sad and embarrassed," she says. "I didn't tell people I had gestational diabetes."

Women who have gestational diabetes often have larger babies and added health concerns—especially if it isn't well-managed—so Mladenovsky decided to switch from a midwife to an obstetrician, who assured her that everything would be okay. She was also referred to an endocrinologist and had biweekly appointments to monitor her blood sugar, diet, weight, and blood pressure. She took nightly insulin and struggled with figuring out the right dosages, but she was determined to get everything right to ensure a healthy pregnancy.

Since then, she hasn't had much follow-up in regard to her diabetes. She went for a six-week checkup to determine that the diabetes had gone away post-pregnancy, but otherwise, she didn't receive a lot in the way of support or information about her future risk.

Tanya Rutley of Victoria, B.C., reports the same. "My health care team mostly discussed type 2 diabetes risk with me and instructed me to continue similar activity and eating habits to reduce the risk, and I'll have to go in for a screening every few years," she says.

Like Mladenovsky, Rutley was diagnosed at 27 weeks. It was her second pregnancy, and she had not developed gestational diabetes the first time around. She found the experience very stressful, as she dealt with blood sugar spikes every morning, despite following all the advice on how to avoid them. She was vigilant about exercise and eating and learned a lot about not just what to eat but also how to pair foods correctly to get the most benefit from nutrition and avoid blood sugar fluctuations.

"This was a huge learning curve, and honestly, while I'd rather not have gestational diabetes, I'm a bit glad I did, as it forced me to eat healthy and consciously. As far as the actual pregnancy, the most impact it had on me was on how and when I gave birth. At around 38 weeks, my numbers started to plummet. Because of this, I had to be induced and gave birth ten days early," she says.

Rutley has a family history of diabetes, so her risk of developing gestational diabetes was higher than the average. Even knowing this and understanding that it was partially genetic, she was devastated by the diagnosis. "I felt like having gestational diabetes was entirely my fault. I should have been eating better, exercising more. I *did this* to my baby," she says now. "My nurse and dietician were amazing, though. They were incredibly reassuring and informative and always available to help me with any questions or concerns I had. I think my gestational diabetes journey would have been much more difficult if it wasn't for these two incredible women." Rutley, who delivered a healthy baby girl, Estie, did not have diabetes post-pregnancy. She shared her experience with gestational diabetes via Instagram, giving a voice to a very common diagnosis that is often mired in shame for those who have it.

"When I got the news, I felt completely alone, shocked, and like it was all my fault. I wanted to reach out to others who might have gone through it and learn through their experiences. The more I learned, the more I realized how misunderstood gestational diabetes is, so I started to share my journey so others could learn from it," she says. "If someone else starting their own gestational diabetes journey came across those posts, then all the better. It was a great outlet, as moms who've gone through it helped me immensely by sharing their experiences, giving information, and making me feel more informed and not alone."

Rutley definitely would have taken a program like the one Lipscombe is piloting if it had been offered. "In all honesty, I have had a hard time keeping up with the lifestyle post-pregnancy. I try to pair carbs with a protein as much as possible, but I'm not as strict as before, nor am I as active," she says. "Of course, when you're pregnant, the effects of gestational diabetes are that much more immediate, whereas the possibility of getting type 2 seems far off and nonthreatening. If I had a team to coach me through it, much like my gestational diabetes team did, it would help keep me accountable."

This accountability is a big part of the process, but it's also a challenging one. In addition, there's a concern that some doctors aren't explaining the future risks well enough when a patient is told their blood sugars have returned to normal. One of Lipscombe's students actually made this suggestion to her as they pondered the question as to why more women don't sign up for available interventions or even look for them. Perhaps when a doctor tells a new mom that their blood tests are back in a normal range, she sees the threat as no longer imminent and moves on to more pressing concerns—like her new baby.

"It's a mixed message," Lipscombe says. "More and more of our diabetes teams are counselling women about the implications for a mother's health long term, but my experience being a clinician is that this kind of message is very hard for women to hear when they are so focused on their baby."

There are some programs that start the intervention earlier—during pregnancy—but she is concerned that the stress of checking blood sugars four times a day, as needed for someone with gestational diabetes, and the worry that any deviation to this will harm their babies, is already enough for a woman dealing with the seemingly endless medical appointments, classes, and other preparations that come with pregnancy. Adding one more intervention might just be too overwhelming, and it may be the item that women choose to skip on an already overly long list.

＊ ＊ ＊ ＊ ＊

While Lipscombe's made-in-Canada program is supporting women who have had gestational diabetes, what about those who already have diabetes when they become pregnant? This is an area that Toronto's Dr. Denice Feig is extremely passionate about. The endocrinologist and diabetes researcher at Mount Sinai's Leadership Sinai Centre for Diabetes started seeing patients with gestational diabetes early in her career and soon began to specialize in the area of diabetes and pregnancy. She is now one of the top researchers in the field internationally.

For a woman diagnosed with type 1 diabetes in childhood or young adulthood, pregnancy is something that weighs heavily on their mind as they mature. Diabetes and pregnancy come with an enormous amount of uncertainty and stress because of the unique challenges and risk of complications. And as type 2 diabetes is being diagnosed in younger and younger women, physicians have to look at how to ensure they have healthy babies, too.

"It's very important for women with type 1 and type 2 diabetes to plan their pregnancies, because if they enter pregnancy and have high blood sugars during the first trimester, then the baby can have an increased risk of birth defects," explains Feig. "If, however, they plan their pregnancy and their blood sugars are good going into pregnancy, then the chance of a birth defect is very similar to the general population. But this is difficult to achieve."

There are many reasons why it can be challenging to keep blood sugars stable during pregnancy. Not least of which is that it's already incredibly difficult to keep them stable when your body isn't going through the process of growing a human. Stress can also have an enormous impact on blood sugar control, and pregnancy can be very stressful in and of itself—especially for women who must be so incredibly vigilant about their health.

Feig has seen many women in her practice who are struggling with these concerns, and it fuels her work. "I think women are afraid that they can't have a healthy baby, but I'd like to let them know that if they plan a pregnancy, then many times we have excellent outcomes," she says, stressing again how critical it is to have a health care team that understands the challenges and can support a mother-to-be throughout her pregnancy.

When my colleague Pilar was pregnant, she felt this stress acutely. Diagnosed with type 1 diabetes at age nineteen, Pilar was well-aware of the risks as she planned her pregnancy. She needed to get permission from a host of health care professionals, she notes, as they signed off on her body's readiness to accomplish what for many women just comes naturally. It wasn't easy, but her first pregnancy was a success, and she felt more confident when she started planning for her second.

But as with any pregnancy, what went well the first time around doesn't always work so well the second time. Pilar struggled with her blood sugar levels, and the stress of this was extremely challenging. She ended up having to take an abrupt and early maternity leave, and her second daughter's birth was complicated.

"The second pregnancy brought much more stress. My blood sugars were better in my first pregnancy, but not because I wasn't as diligent, it was because there was a lack of time and increased stress levels," she explains. Being a full-time working mother to a toddler while managing a second pregnancy with type 1 diabetes was much more challenging.

"In the first pregnancy, all I had to do was focus on myself. I could sleep when I wanted, eat when I wanted, and just focus on the pregnancy and blood sugars, in addition to the rest of my life. In the second pregnancy, the stress was astronomical. I was near a mental breakdown, as I couldn't deal with work, being pregnant, the diabetes, and a small child who needed me all the time. The stress made my blood sugars go up, and I was urged by my medical team to stop working."

While Pilar pushed to stay at work for as long as she could, her medical team finally ordered her to stop. It was just too risky for the baby. The whole pregnancy, she admits, was tough. "I was very concerned about what was happening to her," she says of the little girl growing inside her. "It made me feel guilty. I was scared of what was going to happen, how she would turn out. At times, it made me regret my decisions about having a second child."

The risks of high blood sugar levels during pregnancy are clear, but it's an intense balancing act to try and avoid the stress that can skyrocket your blood sugar levels while at the same time worrying that you are going to have high blood sugar that harms your baby.

"The physical portion of pregnancy is hard, but it doesn't compare to the mental anguish felt by women living with type 1 diabetes who are pregnant," says Pilar. "The guilt eats you up. Wakes you in the night. Haunts your every meal. Knowing that you could possibly harm your unborn child is not something that is easy to explain." Having her children, though, has been an incredible gift. "In the end, it's all worth it."

Feig's research aims to change things for moms-to-be with diabetes. Her goal is to find ways to make pregnancy less stressful and more medically stable. Towards that end, she led the CONCEPTT Trial, which looked at the use of continuous glucose monitoring (CGM) in pregnant women with type 1 diabetes. CGM is a newer technology, which a person wears on their body, typically in the form of a patch. It constantly reads their blood sugar levels and can quickly alert the wearer to fluctuations. For a woman who is going through pregnancy, it can be game-changing.

"The trial found that women with type 1 diabetes using continuous glucose monitoring had markedly improved fetal outcomes, decreased ICU admissions over 24 hours, decreased large babies, and decreased neonatal hypoglycemia," says Feig.

This outcome is an important one, as it shows the potential for CGM to have positive impacts. It has also inspired other researchers, including Cambridge University's Dr. Helen Murphy, to look at closed-loop solutions—meaning that the CGM would monitor blood sugars and then inform the wearer's insulin pump to provide the needed amount of insulin to achieve optimal blood sugar levels. Even just ten years ago, the idea of a completely automated system to manage diabetes seemed unlikely. Now it seems almost inevitable.

For women like Pilar, this would be a welcome change. Now the mother of two healthy and happy little girls, she has no plans to try for a third but also has no regrets about having gone through the challenges of managing diabetes while pregnant. She does, however, stress that she could not have done it without the team of health care professionals that coached her through the process. "I would not have been able to do this without the support of my amazing diabetes educator and endocrinologist. They were my lifelines," she says. "Without them, I literally don't think I could have done it."

Physician-scientists like Lipscombe, Retnakaran, and Feig are just a handful of the Canadian researchers making remarkable progress in the area of women and diabetes. Their work is doing much to support the health concerns faced by female patients across the country and to ensure that women like Tara, Pilar, and the others whose stories I've shared can live healthier lives with or without diabetes. Still, as remarkable as all of their work is and as inspired as I am by the promise of it, there's a part of me that can't help but wonder how much further along research in this area would be if the world of medical science had seen the need for female-specific solutions even earlier.

CHAPTER NINE
Family Ties

After I speak to Dr. Kaberi Dasgupta on the phone for the first time, I hang up and tell my colleague that I'd like to be best friends with her. Having spent more time with her since then, the urge remains the same.

Dasgupta, a clinician-scientist at Montréal's McGill University who grew up on Prince Edward Island, has the sort of sunny disposition and easy laughter that makes it hard to resist slipping into a chat with her. The warmth she emits makes you want to tell her all your problems because surely, she can make everything right in the world. These qualities, no doubt, serve her well in her role as a physician and epidemiologist who specializes in researching trends in diabetes.

When I ask her what motivates her, she says as much. As a general internist, she was increasingly interested in type 2 diabetes, mainly because that was the type of diabetes she tended to see most in her patients. Dasgupta wondered why that was and what could be done to change the upward trajectory of the disease. Asking this question, as many a diabetes researcher will tell you, opens up a Pandora's box of seemingly endless queries.

"What I find really fascinating about diabetes is that it's a condition influenced by so many factors," explains Dasgupta, who realized quickly that this was far from just a biological issue. Social environments and cultural contexts play a role in type 2 diabetes rates, intersecting with biology in ways that are complex and challenging. "There is an association with certain ethnocultural groups, for example, like Indigenous peoples, South Asian people, Black North Americans—

and that's not just biology. That's urbanization, that's colonial histories and exploitation, and that's transgenerational impacts on epigenetic programming. It's not enough to say there's more diabetes in the Cree. There's so much more under that."

This interest, like pulling a thread that unspools more and more from the roll as you go, has driven Dasgupta in unusual directions. In general, a researcher will focus on one area of diabetes. Occasionally, the area of focus will meander into another stream, but the core focus remains.

Not so for Dasgupta. At a talk she gives as part of the University of Toronto's Endocrinology Rounds in mid-2019, she likens her work to *The Lord of the Rings* trilogy, explaining that it's taken on three main tenants thus far—gestational diabetes, type 2 diabetes, and most recently, type 1 diabetes. Moving forward, she may need to think of a longer series to use as an analogy, as she is already well into book three of her series and showing no signs of slowing.

"In all three types, there are genetic factors, health behaviour factors, and social and environmental factors, so the issue is really to acknowledge all of them and try to address all of them in a way to either prevent diabetes or make it easier to live with diabetes," she explains.

While each type has very significant differences and causes, she has also come to see that the solutions may be found somewhere amidst their common ground. Dasgupta's work first gained international notice when she took a deep dive into how type 2 diabetes was an issue that affected families. A 2014 study she led revealed your type 2 diabetes risk increased by 26 percent if your spouse had diabetes, and this generated robust media coverage. However, when she looked deeper, wondering if gestational diabetes could also be a link, her work gained even more attention.

The research clearly showed that a woman with gestational diabetes was at higher risk of developing type 2 diabetes, as were her offspring, but what about the father? The risk to mother and child were in part due to biology, which would seem to leave the spouse in the clear. Using database research, which involves looking at thousands of anonymous cases in one geographic area to find patterns, she determined that, in fact, he wasn't. Dasgupta's research looked at more than 75,000 couples in Québec up to twenty years after the initial gestational diabetes diagnosis, though since her study was published, similar results have been found in other geographical areas. She discovered that when compared to those whose partner had not developed gestational diabetes, the incidence of type 2 diabetes was 33 percent greater in men whose partner had gestational diabetes. Type 2 diabetes, it seemed, was most certainly a family affair.

The idea that a spouse, in this case, a father, was also at risk seems reasonable, as families are often eating the same foods and participating in the same activities, but it was a concept that hadn't been deeply considered before, and Dasgupta's 2015 paper in *Diabetes Care* led to worldwide headlines. The extensive coverage opened up important conversations that supported one of her main arguments—that while gestational diabetes takes place in women, it is far from being an issue exclusive to them.

"If someone in our family has diabetes, it's not their problem alone. It's a *family* issue and a family problem—and maybe even more broadly, society's problem," she says. "At minimum, the family has to work together. If the mother with gestational diabetes is being told by her health care team that she needs to increase her fruit and vegetable consumption and take a walk in the evening, it's very helpful if her partner supports her in doing that."

The families who work together, she explains, are the ones who have more success. These are the families that research shows have a better chance of beating the odds and not seeing the development of type 2 diabetes—or at least putting it off until much later in life.

"The women who have had success are the women who tell me that their kids know what's going on, so they encourage them to go together as a family and exercise. Or their partner is on board with the dietary changes and is willing to make some food changes and prepare healthy meals. Because you can't fight against everything, you can't fight against your desire to have one more cookie and sit in front of the TV, as well as having your family amplifying that." This is a theme I often hear as I research the link between gestational diabetes and type 2 diabetes—that a support system is essential to making lifestyle changes. It's understandable. If you are trying to eat healthy, get more exercise, and reduce stress, yet your partner still wants to eat junk food, it's going to be extremely difficult to change. And in houses where healthy habits aren't the norm, there's a higher risk for everyone to develop type 2 diabetes. Thus, the cycle continues.

Like the work of Dr. Lorraine Lipscombe chronicled in Chapter Eight, Dasgupta's role as a clinician fuels her research. Looking at the data to find these trends is one thing but using that information to develop support programs that look at solutions has to follow. "I think, for me, the importance of any study I do, whether it's a large-scale epidemiological study, a survey, or an intervention, my hope is that it has an importance beyond a published paper or an interesting fact," says Dasgupta. "Knowledge for knowledge's sake is good, but because I am a clinician, I like to know that it has had a concrete effect."

This has led to Dasgupta's work in developing programs to support families who have had gestational diabetes. It has also fueled her continued database research projects, including a 2019 study that once again generated headlines. Having looked at the risks involved when a mother has gestational diabetes, Dasgupta decided to look at the children. That the offspring of mothers with gestational diabetes have a higher likelihood of type 2 diabetes is well-established, but Dasgupta wondered about their future risk for other conditions. She also looked again at their diabetes risk—and was very surprised to see not only the expected increase in type 2 diabetes development but also type 1 diabetes.

Long thought to be an autoimmune disorder, type 1 diabetes typically manifests in childhood or young adulthood and has no known link with lifestyle. To see it showing up more frequently in mothers with gestational diabetes was puzzling. Some have suggested it could be due to exposure to high sugar levels in utero or even the insulin treatment that some mothers receive to treat their gestational diabetes. Whatever the case, Dasgupta is quick to point out that the increase is small—4.52 people per 10,000—but it still gave her pause to consider how this could be translated in a helpful way.

When I attend a presentation on her research, an endocrinologist in the audience asks the same question I have after hearing these conclusions. "This is interesting, but it's also rare, so how do we give this information to women with gestational diabetes without creating unnecessary worry?"

When I speak with her afterwards, Dasgupta agrees that the risk is small—but also important. She tells me a story about when her family was visiting Chile years ago. Her youngest son was still little and, as she watched him play on the beach near the Pacific, she pictured him being pulled in by the waves. This fleeting thought prepared her when, moments later, she found herself bounding into the water after him. Her son was fine, and her quick actions and an older cousin blocking the water ensured he wasn't pulled in fully, but the experience stuck with her. Later, she read research that talked about this phenomenon, where parents tend to react faster when they have thought about a situation before.

"You don't want to create anxiety or paranoia because that's not helpful to anyone," she says. "But the parent had imagined the scenario in his or her head a few times, so when the situation happened, it wasn't out of the blue. 'What's happening now?' becomes 'This is truly happening now, and now I'm going to react.' Yes, type 1 diabetes is rare, and nothing any parent should have to deal with when their child develops it, so knowing that it's possible and how to react if it happens—just as you know your child could run across the street into traffic—you stay aware and vigilant when there's traffic around."

Dasgupta's foray into type 1 diabetes could be unsteady ground for a researcher whose interests have been primarily in gestational and type 2 diabetes, but her work had previously led her into interesting territory with type 1 and established her as a positive force for that community.

In trying to break down barriers and establish better supports for both women with gestational diabetes and patients with type 2 diabetes, she has also encountered a number of people with type 1 diabetes who felt significant stress and stigma around their disease. Type 2 diabetes is often associated with lifestyle, which plays a role, though it's far more complicated than that. Type 1 diabetes, in contrast, has no lifestyle connection.

The constant confusion by the general public about the differences between type 1 and type 2 diabetes doesn't help. People with type 1 often felt that they were being blamed for having a disease that they could not have prevented, and this has led to deep feelings of anxiety and resentment. This in turn led some—in particular young people—to try to hide their condition, which then leads to poorly managed blood sugars and an increased risk of complications later in life.

"Addressing the feeling of stigma and making environments less stigmatizing has the potential to not only let people feel better in general, but specifically improve their blood sugar control, reduce their risk of low blood sugars, and help prevent the complications of diabetes," Dasgupta explains. While this is true of all forms of diabetes, her team was particularly interested in young people with type 1—those who are known for having the most difficult time managing their A1Cs and who have the most to lose if their management is poor.

Dasgupta had a key ally in her foray into type 1 diabetes. Montréal researcher Dr. Anne-Sophie Brazeau had recently taken on a postdoctoral position in Dasgupta's lab. Brazeau had previously worked as a hospital dietitian with a focus on patients with diabetes, helping them manage the complicated carb counting and food decisions they needed to make to maintain good blood sugar control. This led to her interest in pursuing a PhD in the area, which she completed under the mentorship of Dr. Rémi Rabasa-Lhoret at Université de Montréal. Rabasa-Lhoret, a leading expert in type 1 diabetes, had further fueled Brazeau's deep interest in the area of study and also inspired her to look for a postdoctoral position that could expand her knowledge further.

Brazeau had planned to leave Montréal to find her new lab but decided to take another look at the research being done in the city where she had deep roots before she made a decision. There is a bit of a disconnect between the French and English research communities in Québec, and she wondered if perhaps there was work being done in diabetes that she had not yet heard about because of this divide. It turns out, there was—Dasgupta's.

"I was on the McGill website, and I went on her page and went, 'Oh my God, she's doing exactly the kind of research that I was doing, but not with the same population.' I was mainly working with people with type 1 diabetes, and she was working mainly with people with type 2 and gestational diabetes, so I thought it would be a perfect fit."

Brazeau felt that her area of expertise would be an excellent counterbalance to Dasgupta's, and their first meeting confirmed they would be a good match. Dasgupta's enthusiasm immediately resonated with Brazeau, who shares the same exuberance as her mentor, and she started her post-doc position in Dasgupta's lab shortly after the birth of her first child in 2013.

When Dasgupta heard about a funding opportunity for a diabetes stigma project, she asked Brazeau for her thoughts, and the two scientists quickly decided they liked the idea of looking at stigma in youth and young adults who lived with type 1 diabetes. They reached out to youth with type 1, focusing on those aged 14 to 24, and asked them about their experience with stigma. They had 380 respondents— about 65 percent of whom reported feeling stigmatized because of their diabetes. Dasgupta and Brazeau also learned that there was a correlation between blood sugar control and feelings of stigma in those that responded.

"What we've learned is that there's a real need to address stigma in this age group, where people are making career choices, romantic choices, leaving their parents' home to go study elsewhere or live independently, and on top of that, they also have to manage their type 1 diabetes, so that's challenging," Dasgupta says.

Simply identifying a problem has never been satisfying to either Dasgupta or Brazeau, so they took the feedback they received from their initial respondents and looked at what they could do to help. "We asked them, 'What can society do to help you deal with your diabetes?' and one of the comments was that they needed peer support," says Brazeau. "We said, 'OK, now that we know that, we need to propose something.' We cannot just find that there's a gap; we need to fill that gap."

In speaking with young people with type 1 diabetes, the team worked to develop a support system that was sustainable and effective. Through this process, the Virtual Peer Network (VPN) program was developed. An online community currently housed on Facebook, the VPN is a place where those living with type 1 diabetes between the ages of 14 and 24 can connect, share stories, ask questions, and receive the type of peer support that can make them feel more empowered in their management of the condition.

When I meet with a group of young peer support members in the fall of 2017, they are eager to share their commitment to the program. Type 1 diabetes, they explain, is often a hidden disease. You can't look at other people and tell whether or not they have it. It's also rare compared to other chronic health conditions. You may be quite easily the only person in your school or community living with the disease.

* * * * *

I think of this when out with my friend Grace one afternoon. We order lunch at a restaurant, along with diet sodas. A few sips in, Grace expresses concern that this isn't, in fact, diet. Though the waitress assures us it is, a few minutes later Grace pulls out her test kit to check her blood sugar. A regular soda is an annoyance for someone with type 1, but it is fairly easy to deal with when you feel comfortable doing so. When Grace was a teenager in school, where none of her peers had diabetes, she may have felt less comfortable testing in public, leading to a potentially high blood sugar—and the complications that come with it.

For the youth participating in the peer support group, the idea is to make these types of situations less fraught. A young adult can coach a teenager through the difficult transitions and help them feel empowered and supported. Is it the answer to the complex question of how to ease transitions from pediatric to adult care in type 1 diabetes? No. But it's a step in the right direction.

The group can also help with education, something that is much needed to help the public better understand the differences between type 1 and type 2 diabetes. "There are similarities, and there are differences," explains Dasgupta. "While both have high blood sugar levels, in type 2, if one is able to change their eating patterns and physical activity, we can change the need for medication, and often pills may be adequate, whereas, in type 1, it's insulin from the outset. And the physical activity and eating *are* important, but they're not going to be the exclusive solution. People with type 1 have to navigate a very narrow space between lows and highs, which makes the challenge all the more difficult."

The confusion between the different types of diabetes comes up frequently enough for those that work in diabetes research that you will find most walk a tightrope in terms of trying to use the correct distinction at all times. In my own work hosting the *Diabetes Canada Podcast*, I have tried to do the same—always clarifying what someone is talking about. The most mortifying moment for me was listening to one of my podcasts and realizing I had mistakenly said type 2 when I meant type 1. It seems like a little thing, but for those living with the condition, the stigma around type 2 diabetes (whether it is deserved or not) comes up so often as a source of stress that it's difficult not to feel concerned that you may have contributed to this negative feeling.

"I think what people with type 1 get frustrated with is when it's assumed that they have their condition because they didn't eat well," says Dasgupta, expressing one of the most common misconceptions about the disease. She is quick to note that there is an extensive stigma and misunderstanding around type 2 diabetes, as well, which is one of the things that makes this work particularly challenging. While it is often associated with lifestyle and obesity, the actual root causes are much more complex. "I'm working at the same time in different types of diabetes: type 2 diabetes, gestational diabetes, and type 1 diabetes. And even though those are all different and affect different groups of people, they have some commonalities because it's hard to manage a chronic disease. And in diabetes, you always have to be watching what you're eating and how you're being physically active, as well as taking your medications."

The common thread that sews each of Dasgupta's projects together has been the role of family and connections, be they others with the same disease or those inside their household. This helps us understand the development of diabetes and the supports needed for those who have it, or in the case of type 2 diabetes, those trying to prevent it.

Dasgupta, in her sunny, charming way, is perhaps the perfect person to attempt to bridge these gaps and create these connections. It's hard not to be swayed by her energy and optimism, particularly since it sits alongside a deep intelligence and is backed by extensive data.

Brazeau would agree. "She always finds the positive side of everything, so it's a pure joy to work with her," she says of her mentor, noting that Dasgupta will fight to fund research she feels will help people and then continue to fight to implement change based on her findings. "Whether the results are positive or negative, it's not the end. After that, we need to make sure there's a real knowledge transfer so that other people know about this."

Diabetes, whatever the type, is a real challenge, and Dasgupta sees research as a way to help people overcome these obstacles. Her work in chronic disease has shown that when people are given the tools, and the barriers are reduced, true change is possible.

"The knowledge comes from the study, and the inspiration comes from the individual patients," she explains. "I think the truth is that when you watch people live with a chronic disease like diabetes, that in itself is quite encouraging. But I am also inspired by the way that people will engage when I work with them."

In speaking about one of her prevention programs for type 2 diabetes, she makes an analogy that seems applicable to all of her various projects. "What was motivating was how engaged people were with a small, simple intervention, and how willing people often are to improve their health with the right mix of support from their health care teams, their families, and society as a whole. I think just as we develop some forms of diabetes incrementally over time, or our risk for them, the solutions can also be small steps that get us to the right place."

CHAPTER TEN

Welcome to the Neighbourhood

When Dr. Gillian Booth steps on stage as a keynote speaker at the 2019 Diabetes Canada Professional Conference in Winnipeg, Manitoba, the room is full. It's a testament to her and how much the type of research she does has been accepted. Back in the day, many scientists pooh-poohed the idea of looking at trends in population health or health services. They didn't believe it could have a real impact on diabetes and other chronic illnesses.

Booth, her red hair in a sleek bob, finds her stride as the slides unfurl before her. She is here to talk about how the social and environmental determinants of health—where you live, what you have access to, and how much money you have—have a real impact on your type 2 diabetes risk. Her work has garnered worldwide attention. In particular, her studies about how living in a walkable community can decrease a person's chances of developing type 2 diabetes. The audience listens attentively as she presents new data about other impacts, as well—everything from air pollution to housing insecurity.

Her final slide elicits the strongest applause as Booth displays a photo of her mentor, Dr. Jan Hux, and talks about the impact Hux has had not only on her career—but on this entire field of science. It was Hux who first used Ontario's health data to track diabetes in the province, which in turn has helped improve how the condition is managed. Hux, who went on to become the president and CEO of Diabetes Canada, and who, in full disclosure, has also been a mentor to me in my career, announced that she would step down from her role in January 2020. Her impending retirement and what that would mean for the Canadian diabetes research landscape was on the minds of everyone in the room during Booth's touching tribute.

When Hux began her research career in 1992, it was impossible to imagine that epidemiology and population study in the diabetes space would one day be featured on the plenary stage of Canada's largest and most influential diabetes conference. Now, it seems impossible to consider that it wouldn't—and to have one of her star mentees giving the presentation makes the moment so much sweeter.

As a clinician, Hux initially focused entirely on seeing patients. Over time, though, she began to wonder if there was a way she could have a larger and deeper impact on the care that people received. "It is such a privilege to connect with patients and families at the time of illness and to bring that care and understanding—even in situations where there's not a lot you can do to change the course of the illness," she says. "To further understanding and communicate a path forward can bring great reassurance and comfort to people. That's such rewarding work. Every day you feel appreciated and see an opportunity to make a difference, and you're impacting people one by one by one. Even though I loved that work, I moved on to something else because I wanted to not just impact people individually—but populations."

With a Master's degree in epidemiology from the Harvard School of Public Health, Hux developed expertise in looking at chronic disease through the lens of populations. She brought that experience to her work at the Institute for Clinical Evaluative Sciences (ICES), where she was first a trainee, then a scientist, and later Deputy CEO. ICES is a not-for-profit research institute with a focus on using Ontario health and patient administrative data—such as Ontario Health Insurance Plan (OHIP) records— to study health-related issues. With her interest in taking a population focus, it was a perfect fit for Hux.

Her biggest breakthrough, she admits, "is a story of success born out of failure." Hux had just earned a faculty position at the University of Toronto and had written her first grant. She asked for a fairly small sum to use the administrative data available through ICES to map the diabetes epidemic in Ontario. She was excited about the project and felt it was an easy win. The number of people in the province living with diabetes was information Ontario didn't have but sorely needed.

And then she didn't get the grant. Her reviewers felt she wouldn't be able to use the administrative databases to get the information she wanted and that there was too high a likelihood that her data sources would misidentify people as having diabetes, thereby skewing the results.

Hux disagreed, but she didn't know what to do next. She was sitting in her office considering the problem when Dr. Vivek Goel dropped by to chat. Listening to her dilemma, he suggested that she go back and ask for a lot more money, so she could actually get the information she needed to confirm whether or not you can accurately identify people with diabetes using administrative records. If the reviewers didn't think it was possible, then she needed to undertake this much larger project to show them it was.

And so that's exactly what she did. This time not only did she receive the grant, but she now had the funds to expand the project scope to show that not only was the information there but that it could be used to better inform health care policy. Hux was also able to get permission from the Privacy Commissioner of Ontario to use primary patient medical records to confirm if someone had diabetes or not and to correlate this back to the administrative data available through OHIP records.

Hux developed a system modelled on a similar one researchers in Manitoba had used, which would consider someone as having diabetes if there had been two or more notes from a physician made in their records or if they had one hospitalization for diabetes. The project, she admits, was not the sort of exciting science some people envision. Her team spent a lot of time visiting primary care doctors and pulling charts, flipping through vast amounts of paperwork to find the pieces she needed. An enormous amount of time was spent crunching the numbers she found. But in the end, it was an incredible success.

"We were actually picking out 86 percent of [diabetes] cases," Hux explains. "And the misclassification—labelling someone as having diabetes when they didn't—was less than three percent. So we were really confident then to use that data to map the diabetes epidemic."

This new algorithm had an enormous impact on the research landscape in Canada. Since it was first published, it has been used widely, and many other researchers have adopted her process—with excellent results. According to Google Scholar, which tracks the citations for scientific papers, Hux's has been cited more than a thousand times—an impressive achievement for a researcher in any field.

Along the way, Hux began to mentor other female physicians and scientists who were interested in pursuing health services research. Mentorship was important to her, as she had few role models growing up. "I didn't go to med school until I was 29, in part because I couldn't see myself as a career person," she says. "I grew up in this small farming community. Neither of my parents finished high school, and the jobs that were available to women were store clerk, secretary, or elementary school teacher, and none of those really appealed to me."

Hux admits she felt a bit lost before she started medical school, but it was through her work in health care that she found support. As she began to take on her own students, she wanted to ensure they were better equipped to navigate the complexities of science. She was also passionate about being able to integrate the challenges of motherhood into a career that is not always easy for those who want to raise children.

There is a nurturing quality to Hux, a trait that no doubt served her well as a physician, but which also makes her particularly well suited to be a mentor. I have joked with her a few times that her superpower is her ability to make me cry—not in a bad way—because she just seems to have an innate talent for listening and understanding in a way that can break down emotional walls. She can also showcase a steely willpower and determination in the face of adversity, in addition to her analytical and brilliant mind, and this has helped make her a respected and beloved champion for people living with diabetes—and for those who want to develop treatments and cures.

Hux had hoped to have a family of her own, but she found her person, her late husband Edwin, later in life, and instead, she slipped easily into the role of a devoted stepmother and grandmother. Scientists like Booth and Lipscombe have become a second family of sorts. In them, Hux found students and people who are as talented and passionate about their work as she is. She has pushed them as researchers and nurtured them as people, imparting on them her scientific acumen and her belief in the importance of empathy.

Lipscombe credits a study she and Hux published in the prestigious academic journal, *The Lancet,* as a pivotal point in her career. Looking at data regarding the diabetes rates in Ontario, the researchers saw a sharp increase in type 2 diabetes rates in the province. Lipscombe wondered if there was a way to highlight how substantial this increase was by looking at it through an epidemiological and population lens. Hux encouraged her to be creative. While a relative increase of 70 percent over ten years seemed substantial enough on its own, the scientists were well aware that this type of story had been told many times in the media—and without context, it often failed to resonate. "I had a lightbulb moment, and I thought, well, have people made any predictions? What did people think was going to happen?"

Digging into the data, Lipscombe found that, yes, there were predictions available. A World Health Organization study had predicted the rate of diabetes would go up by about 30 percent by 2020. That Ontario had already reached that number in 2005 and was projected to greatly surpass it by 2020 was just the angle the story needed.

Lipscombe looked at the data to determine how the rates were growing in different age groups and if there were any trends amongst the population that were statistically significant. She considered mortality rates among the population, and by scouring all of the information available, she was able to frame her career-making paper, which has gone on to influence public policy thinking on diabetes in the province.

Hux, she notes, encouraged her to follow her instincts and work on projects that resonated with her while also mentoring her on the complexities of being a woman in science. Especially one working in the area of health services research, which was still facing skepticism from the basic and clinical research communities. While epidemiology has been an ongoing force in research, the idea of studying health care data to battle chronic illness was initially met with resistance.

This is no longer the case, and a new wave of health services researchers benefit today from the path Hux and her first wave of students have blazed. Dr. Alanna Weisman, an endocrinologist in Toronto and a rising star in the Canadian diabetes research landscape, is using the databases Hux fought to access and the models Hux and her team proved were effective in order to try and better understand type 1 diabetes. While Hux's work was able to determine overall diabetes rates in the general population, there was no easy way to determine if the patient had type 1 or type 2 diabetes. Since the needs of each population are very different, being able to separate them in the data would be enormously helpful.

"We've been doing research using this type of data in Canada for many years," she says. "Basically, since the '90s, when Jan Hux led the effort to identify who has diabetes in this data. The major limitation was that we couldn't distinguish type 1 diabetes and type 2 diabetes, so it was much harder to study type 1 diabetes because the numbers are much smaller than people with type 2 diabetes, and as a result, we actually knew very little about type 1 diabetes at a population level."

The data available to researchers, which is all de-identified and coded without names, gives them a way to look at populations from a macro level. While it can be fairly easy to see who has diabetes, determining if someone has type 1 or type 2 presents a number of challenges. This is due to the complicated system used to identify conditions in medical records, which in the province of Ontario, as an example, involves different codes used in hospitals versus outpatient care. For a family doctor or specialist working outside a hospital, there is only one billing code for diabetes, whereas in a hospital setting there are many more. So, if a patient is never admitted to a hospital as a result of their diabetes, the type of disease they have may never be accurately captured in the database.

In the past, someone who was diagnosed with diabetes in adolescence likely had type 1, but as an increasing number of people with type 2 are being diagnosed at younger ages. Additionally, type 1 diabetes is often diagnosed in adults. Weisman has worked with Booth to find data points—things like insulin pump use, which is specific to those with type 1, or insulin prescriptions starting at a young age—that allowed them to design an algorithm to better determine who in the population has which type of diabetes.

Weisman uses the databases developed at ICES and the newest resource, the National Diabetes Repository, developed by Diabetes Action Canada, to study access to health care and related outcomes.

"We know a lot about diabetes in Ontario, and a lot of that information is from using these types of data sources. So we can tell you what the number of people with diabetes is, how much these numbers are increasing—or are projected to increase in the future—and how this varies by where someone lives. We know there are areas where the rates of diabetes are much higher than others," Weisman says, highlighting just why it was so important to provide controlled and de-identified access to this data to researchers.

"We really couldn't tell you anything like that about type 1 diabetes. We couldn't tell you [something] as basic as how many people in Ontario have type 1 diabetes, how well are they doing with their diabetes care and controlling blood sugars, and how much is type 1 diabetes costing the health system. We weren't able to answer any of those questions without being able to conduct this kind of research. So I think now because we've just recently been able to make this distinction, we'll be able to inform ourselves so much more about type 1 diabetes in Ontario, and I really think this will improve the care for people with type 1 diabetes, and perhaps also influence how we're delivering health care to them."

Having this kind of data can be enormously helpful for improvements to treatment and care. Insulin pumps, which deliver insulin continuously to a person with diabetes, have been shown, in some cases, to have a positive impact on diabetes management and blood sugar control. These devices are fully covered in some provinces, but not all. Now that Weisman can see who in the population has type 1 diabetes, she can look at things like their rates of hospitalization, diabetic ketoacidosis, and other markers that can show improvements in overall health—and potentially health care savings—in provinces that provide full coverage for pumps. For someone in Manitoba with type 1 diabetes, who as of this writing, does not have coverage past the age of 18, that sort of information could help with advocacy to the government to request better funding.

"We know so little, and there's so much that we'll discover," says Weisman of the work. "Now that we have the opportunity to look at multiple provinces [through the Diabetes Action Canada National Diabetes Repository], we're going to actually see how these funding programs influence insulin pump use, who is using insulin pumps, and whether there is rationale to say that funding for insulin pumps should be available universally across Canada, which it currently isn't in all provinces."

This result—the potential to actually change the health care land-scape for people with diabetes—is one of the most motivating factors for Hux. She cites Weisman's work as a good example of how this type of research can have impact. "The naysayers who think health services research is just bean-counting, they'd say, 'That's not even science. Of course, the people who get pumps are going to do bet-ter because they're better at self-advocacy, they have a stronger social support system, and they're likely more affluent. Whether they had a pump or syringes or were snorting the insulin up their nose, they're going to do better because of those factors.' But good health services researchers will create models where they will actually control for those differences in baseline characteristics. And so really exciting, advanced statistical methods have been developed to deal with those very problems."

This wide lens on trends in populations, and the algorithm Hux developed, are tools Booth also applies to her work. Her influential study on walkability in neighbourhoods won praise from the scientif-ic community and public policymakers when it was released in 2016. It explores how where you live can impact your type 2 diabetes risk in a way that is easy to understand. It also hit home with many people who are looking at how the infrastructure we have created in cities may be having a significant effect on the explosion of new cases of type 2 diabetes in Canada and worldwide. "Our research has focused on how the way we design or structure neighbourhoods can influence your health, particularly, the risk of diabetes and related diseases," Booth explains. In the past, neighbourhoods were often created around pedestrian activity. Now, however, they are often designed around cars. "A lot of the modern suburbs are more sprawling, and they're zoned in such a way that stores and other places you might walk to are not accessible by foot, so you have to get in your car and drive. And that car dependency is really something that has become more of the modern norm."

She set out to determine if this change in how communities are built would make a difference in type 2 diabetes risk—and she found that it did. Her highly regarded 2016 study on this topic was published in *JAMA: The Journal of the American Medical Association*. It looked at the association between neighbourhood walkability and obesity and diabetes and showed that over a 12-year period, those in communities that provided a walkable urban design had a decreased risk of developing type 2 diabetes. These are the sort of stats that make governments and policymakers take notice. In fact, on an episode of the *Diabetes Canada Podcast* in 2017, Dr. Teresa Tam, the Chief Public Health Officer for Canada, cited Booth's study as something governments could look at to enact change.

This work, though, is not so simple as just determining that all cities must now be made walkable, and thus, the type 2 diabetes epidemic is ended. While Booth looks to prove that these elements play a role, she and other researchers know that it's a confluence of many factors that has created the problem we now face.

"I think it's really helpful in developing the whole picture," Booth says. "A lot of research on the built environment has focused on one risk factor at a time. We know that if you live in a walkable community, you're at lesser risk for developing diabetes, but then there's other factors, such as access to fast food, air pollution, and the social structure of neighbourhoods that are also contributing. We need to understand how all of those things together play a role." For instance, what if your walkable community has a great deal of air pollution? That's a question one of her former PhD students, Nick Howell, decided to look at, and his findings are a great example of why population health interventions are so complex.

"If you live in a walkable neighbourhood that has low levels of traffic-related pollution, your risk of diabetes and high blood pressure is quite low, in fact much lower than we would have expected," Booth explains. "But if you live in a walkable neighbourhood where there's lots of traffic-related pollution, you actually don't see any benefit. The advantage you get from walking may be matched by an increased risk of diabetes and high blood pressure associated with air pollution. So, there's a lot of these complexities that we're trying to disentangle."

It's a similar issue when you look at the food environment, which Booth did in 2015. In many places, people live in what is considered a "food desert." These areas offer poor access to healthy and fresh foods. People there are at higher risk for obesity or type 2 diabetes. Booth looked at the research on this topic and wondered if when people are surrounded by a large variety of unhealthy fast-food restaurants, which she deemed "fast-food swamps," the results would show that the availability of these options would impact outcomes.

Her study, which was published in the journal *Preventive Medicine*, looked at the type 2 diabetes risk in people with "fast-food swamps" within a ten-minute walk from their home versus those who lived further from these areas. The results showed that people who live near one of these swamps had a higher risk of developing type 2—even if it was part of a walkable community.

"Being able to walk to places is great, but there's other risks we need to address," Booth says. "One of the big-ticket items we've learned is that the answers and solutions to the problems aren't necessarily straightforward or easy. We know we need to get people moving, but we don't necessarily know the best or most cost-effective way to do that on a population level. When it comes down to the bottom line, there isn't going to be a single answer, but dozens or even hundreds of little things that really need to happen to actually change the way we live our life."

This is at the heart of the prevention puzzle. There have been a number of advances in type 2 diabetes treatments and prevention strategies over the years, but because there are so many moving pieces and potential factors, it's easy to narrow the lens too much or widen it too broadly. Because of this, not everyone benefits from the interventions that are created—often those who are already the most marginalized benefit the least. Looking at potential risk from a population level helps address the root causes while including everyone in the process.

The researchers continuing this work, who are committed to systemic change, inspire Hux as she begins her retirement. Her beloved husband, Edwin, died unexpectedly in 2019, and it changed much about how she viewed her future. Her day-to-day work running Diabetes Canada has been replaced with time spent managing her garlic farm just outside of Toronto, catching up on her knitting, and volunteering with the causes she and Edwin supported.

She remains deeply connected to her children and grandchildren, as well as her extended family of former students. While she has no desire to return to diabetes research, she will still be a mentor and friend to the scientists whose research she has helped shape, and she looks forward to cheering them on from the sidelines. "I feel like that next generation, they have far surpassed me, and I'm absolutely delighted by that. I never made full professor, but I was at Gillian Booth's professor day, and it was such a happy, happy day to see my kids exceed me."

"Home Sweet Home(less)"

The atrium at the Li Ka Shing Knowledge Institute at St. Michael's Hospital in Toronto is not typically the setting for an art exhibit, but as I wander through the photos set up on easels around the sunny space, I am struck by the impact art can have on our understanding of research and of the human condition.

Today I am here to see the culmination of a project coordinated by Dr. David Campbell. Called "Home Sweet Home(less)," the exhibit showcases the experiences of a group of Toronto residents who are living with both homelessness and diabetes. The dozen or so photos on display are stark and powerful, giving visual representation to an experience that I had only understand on a theoretical level before today.

As a medical student in Calgary, Alberta, Campbell had the opportunity to work at and then lead a student-developed program to support the homeless population in the city. It was an experience that changed the way he looked at the health and social issues faced by those who experience housing insecurity.

When he decided to pursue a postdoctoral fellowship, he chose to study under Dr. Gillian Booth in Toronto. The project he proposed was a unique one, and he knew Booth, who has done extensive research into the socioeconomic impacts of diabetes, would be an excellent person to learn from. Campbell proposed that he would talk to those who had experience of living with homelessness and diabetes, so he could better understand the challenges they faced on a daily basis and what they saw as their greatest areas of need.

Homelessness itself can be difficult to define. Campbell points out that many of us consider the homeless to be the people we see sitting on the street corner, asking for change. There are a number of people, though, who cycle through stages of housing instability. They may have unstable employment and have housing while they are working, and then lose it when they are out of work again, or they may be dealing with other issues that cause them to be without housing on a stable basis.

Whatever the situation, Campbell knew that a great number of these people also lived with diabetes—usually type 2. Policymakers and scientists had often suggested solutions that might help with some of the barriers, including difficulty finding consistent care, lack of access to medications, and the ability to take them on a regular basis. Loss of identification cards and inadequate foot care, which leads to increased risk of amputation, were also major concerns. The list was long and seemingly endless. But these were all things developed through the lens of population health—things that were known because the homeless population as a whole had been studied. But if he asked people what *they* saw as their biggest struggle, would their answers line up?

And once he had their answers, how could he deliver the information in a way that would resonate and cut through the noise of all the other well-meaning research in the area of homelessness?

Many assumed Campbell's biggest hurdle would be finding people who would participate in the study, which involved regular meetings with his team over several weeks. Wouldn't those dealing with homelessness have bigger and more important things to deal with than a focus group?

"It's very difficult to say what working with the homeless population is like because there's many different subsets. There's the chronically entrenched homeless population, and many of them struggle with mental health and addiction and have many other priorities on their plate other than participating in a research study," he says. "But by the same token, a lot of them like to share their story and actually jump at the opportunity to have their voice heard.

"I'd say, one of the biggest challenges in working with any vulnerable or socially disadvantaged population is getting all of the ethical clearances in place in order to be able to access the population. The ethics boards are certainly very protective about making sure people aren't exploited or taken advantage of, which is a good thing, but once we've cleared all those hurdles, it actually hasn't been that hard to find people. They have been contacting us, wanting to tell their story and be involved."

Trying to find the right medium to share their experiences, he asked participants to document the things that impacted their ability to manage their diabetes in photographs. The photos they ended up taking, displayed in the gallery as large, framed images, are stark and haunting.

Food figures prominently. Many photos of the meals provided at a shelter or food bank showcase the bland, carbohydrate-heavy, highly-processed, sugar-saturated foods people with diabetes are cautioned to avoid. Looking at an image, I feel shaken by my own privilege. I can choose to eat a bowl of corn flakes or a chocolate chip cookie if I want, knowing that I probably shouldn't because they aren't the healthiest choices. But if I was sitting in a homeless shelter looking at my one meal of the day, could I turn that down simply because I knew it wasn't what was best for my chronic health condition?

The viciousness of the cycle is hard to look away from once you see it. If you are housing insecure and you only have $5 for groceries that week, do you buy the box of $3.99 pizza snacks that will tide you over for four days but which have little nutritional value? Or do you buy the $5 bag of salad that will last for a day or two and leave you feeling hungry? How do you decide? When you are dealing with so many other issues, is this even your biggest priority?

At the exhibit opening, Campbell has invited the photographers to stand next to their work and tell their stories to the guests who attend. I stand back, listening as men and women from all sorts of diverse backgrounds speak about the image they felt most captured their experience with diabetes as someone with lived experience of homelessness. I had thought about all the access to care issues, in-

cluding medications and proper footwear to manage diabetic foot ul-
cers, but yet, as with almost everyone who lives with diabetes, it was
food that stood out at the top of the list for those in the study. This
should not have surprised me, and yet it did.

Campbell has since taken the "Home Sweet Home(less)" exhibit
to many diabetes-related events across Canada, and at each one, it
has elicited an enormous response. When possible, he has attempted
to have at least one of the photographers present to talk about their
photo and the experience of participating in this work

It is a project I find myself discussing more frequently, as well.
When a colleague mentions a new nutritional intervention for diabetes, I now feel compelled to bring up the issue of barriers and privilege. Will this work for some of the population? Potentially. But how
are we addressing it with everyone else?

My response is one that Campbell hopes to see from health care
providers, who often have so many things to manage in a visit that
they don't always consider the circumstances each patient faces. "I
think part of our research project has been to hear these stories and
document people's experiences, just to make other health care providers and the health literature aware of what these people face, and how
difficult it is to manage diabetes in the context of so many barriers."

Campbell successfully completed his postdoctoral fellowship and
returned to the University of Calgary, and a faculty appointment with
an endocrinology medical practice. The people he worked with and
the stories he got to tell through this project will remain with him
all his life. "While we as health care providers often think about the
medical side of diabetes, like complications, A1c's, and health-service
delivery, for patients who live with the disease on a daily basis, these
are not the most impactful things," he says. "Many challenging barriers, like those who experience homelessness, issues like emotional
well-being, and meeting their instrumental needs—like housing and
healthy food—are by far the most pressing concerns. That doesn't
mean that we should ignore diabetes because they have lots of other
things going on, but we need alternative approaches to meet their
needs.

CHAPTER ELEVEN
It's All in Your Head

Watching Dr. Michael Vallis address an audience full of people with diabetes is fascinating. The unassuming psychologist, with his longish brown hair and penchant for dad sweaters, is soft-spoken and warm, yet the crowd seems transfixed as if he were an old-school revival preacher or a self-help guru. There is no huckster undertone to Vallis' presentation, though; he's simply doing something every person with diabetes wishes for—explaining that their feelings, stress, and sense of being overwhelmed is normal.

At the end of one presentation, a woman in the crowd stands up to ask whether the Halifax-based therapist would consider taking a patient in Toronto. It's a question on the minds of many in the room, who loudly express their approval at the idea. It's understandable, as Vallis is one of the still far-too-few researchers looking into the area of diabetes and mental health, and his work has highlighted the vast need for more of these services.

Vallis did not intend to spend his career working with people with diabetes. However, after several years working at the Clarke Institute of Psychiatry (now the Centre for Addiction and Mental Health), he applied for and received a position at Mississauga's Credit Valley Hospital. He initially counselled patients managing gastrointestinal issues, then found many diabetes patients were being referred to him, too, as they struggled to cope with the ongoing stress of managing the disease. It was in this setting that he discovered he enjoyed the teamwork aspect of diabetes care teams, and the willingness the found there to consider the psychological impact of illness. He also learned that while psychologists are often focused on helping patients overcome a mood or feeling that is outside of the norm and causing distress, the patents he was seeing who were living with chronic disease did not fall into that category. "When I started to work with patients, what I discovered is that the story they told me actually made perfect sense, and psychopathology doesn't make sense," he says. "I kept thinking, if I was in your situation, and I experienced exactly what you told me, I think I'd feel the exact same way."

This aha moment was so powerful that he moved his practice away from psychopathology and into behaviour. "With chronic disease and chronic conditions, much of what people experience is not their fault. It's not a weakness on their part or pathological on their part. So the focus isn't really on 'We've got to make you change.' It's about 'How do we help you adapt to the situation you're in?' That's kind of the way I fell into diabetes."

Through his work, Vallis found that people with diabetes were desperate for someone to listen to them, someone who would actually understand the reality they faced. Living every day with a disease that offers no vacations and no breaks from day-to-day management is difficult. The fact that it comes with enormous consequences if managed poorly makes it even more distressing. And while it has been known for decades that people with diabetes have higher rates of depression and anxiety, there was little acknowledgement of how those conditions could be completely unique for someone with diabetes.

During her work with Diabetes Canada, Dr. Jan Hux saw firsthand the same things Vallis was observing in his practice. "Diabetes is a 24/7 condition from the time you're diagnosed, and at this point, since we don't have a cure, for the rest of your life. That really takes a toll," she says. "Little, daily decisions can have a huge impact on downstream physical health. Knowing that that failure to exercise or that increase in consumption of ice cream may be the straw that breaks the camel's back and leads to blindness or kidney failure, that's a tremendous amount of pressure to live under, and that impacts people. They feel burdened by the weight of future consequences making their current decisions."

It wasn't until 2005, with the publication of the Diabetes Attitudes, Wishes, and Needs (DAWN) Study, that the idea of "diabetes distress" or a specific form of diabetes-related anxiety became part of popular understanding. Vallis was intrigued by this research, and he started including it in his practice and in his teaching. When a second DAWN Study was announced—DAWN2—the researchers involved were aware of his interest and asked him to represent Canada on the team.

His contribution to that landmark study has been considerable, and his passion for disseminating the findings across the country runs deep. For Vallis, understanding and managing the psychological aspects of diabetes is critical to improving care and making life better for the millions of people living with the disease worldwide.

"It's opened the door. There are now three legitimate diabetes psychological experiences that cannot be ignored by diabetes providers because of the DAWN," Vallis says.

The first of these is "diabetes distress," which is separate from depression or anxiety and which acknowledges that most of the anxiety patients experience is actually related to their disease. The second is a fear of hypoglycemia—or having low blood sugar. Low blood sugars can cause dizziness, an inability to think straight, slurring of words, loss of consciousness, seizures and even—in extreme cases—death. For someone with diabetes, the constant fear that you will go low can be debilitating.

The third is "psychological insulin resistance." This condition, common in those with type 2 diabetes, is tied to the idea that starting insulin is a failure. Vallis has seen through his studies that patients who started insulin in order to lower their A1C results instead found that their numbers rose. "It was like, hang on, how can that be? We got people started on insulin, and yet their A1C control got poorer," he says. "We could get them started, but they wouldn't change the dose, and they wouldn't titrate because of the fear."

This type of problem could likely be mitigated by better explaining that diabetes is a progressive disease when people are diagnosed with type 2. Instead, patients often leave their doctor's office with a prescription for metformin and an understanding that if they take better care of themselves, they can stave off insulin. This is rarely true, no matter how much you adjust your lifestyle, and thinking you have failed when you are prescribed insulin can be a huge emotional blow.

Vallis has already started to see changes in how endocrinologists and family doctors are explaining the progressive nature of type 2 diabetes, following recent studies that highlight how much better people self-manage when they understand that thorough ongoing improvement is needed. "Educating people at the beginning that sometime in the future someone is going to raise the issue of insulin with you. You want to be prepared for that. Because if someone says, 'Oh, yeah, my doctor told me when I was diagnosed that this was probably going to happen, I guess I'm OK with that.' As opposed to, 'I'm a failure,' or 'This is punishment.'"

Much of the work Vallis does is helping explain things like this to health care providers, who are typically treating patients with a condition they themselves don't live with. When starting insulin, for example, doctors have been trained to see this as a positive thing—a way to help their patient improve their blood sugar control and avoid complications from a disease that is very often progressive, regardless of the patient's abilities to adapt to lifestyle changes. It's important to reframe their thinking so they can place themselves in the shoes of their patient, who may interpret starting insulin as a sign they are not self-managing well enough.

It's the same when providers talk about A1Cs in people with both type 1 and type 2 diabetes. Blood sugar levels are one of the most anxiety-producing topics for people living with the disease. Over and over in my own career working in diabetes, I have heard patients tell me how much they hate going to their endocrinologist and having to face a discussion about their A1Cs. They feel like they have failed when their numbers are not good, and they fear that even if they have had mostly good control, their physician will hit on the one or two times when their sugar levels were off-kilter. They also believe their doctor is only interested in the number on their chart—not the myriad reasons they may be struggling with their A1Cs.

People with diabetes want their health care providers to understand their whole life experience because this is critical to successful A1C management. Stress, physical activity, illness, and changes to schedules or sleep patterns—almost everything people experience in day-to-day life can impact someone's A1C levels. Yet there is rarely the opportunity to discuss these factors with the person who's monitoring the numbers.

"Not enough time is spent on that link, which has to do more with listening than it does with speaking, and that's what health care providers can be challenged to do—really *listen*," says Vallis. "I think the answer is that we need to really shift and recognize that chronic disease management is all about the listening and the integration of the person."

The argument is often made that there isn't time in an appointment to include a discussion of the patient's life experience. Doctors, and in particular family practitioners, don't have time to hear a person's whole story in the span of a 15-minute appointment. But those who have studied this area feel like there is a lack of understanding of what it means to have these types of discussions. It doesn't need to be a deep dive into someone's entire life, but the possible improvement in care when the patient's voice is heard is worth making an effort.

Vallis suggests starting an appointment by taking a few minutes to focus on this. "It's really important that we meet your needs. Can we have a conversation about what your needs are, and then perhaps what my interests are? And then would it be OK if we took the first five minutes of the appointment and say, 'I'd like to just listen to you and know what's going on in your life that's relevant to your diabetes,'" Vallis says of the discussion he suggests physicians have. "If you can frame that up in five minutes, then we could say what needs to happen in that session. And I'd be curious: What if we organized our services like that, so it always began with the person able to tell their story?"

Vallis also thinks that this would take the edge off for some doctors, who often feel like the villain in the diabetes story. "I'll say to a physician, 'Does it bother you that your patient thinks you're controlling and judgemental? And the doctor says, 'That's really upsetting to me. I don't want my patients to think I'm controlling and dismissive, and that I'm acting like Atilla the Hun with them,'" Vallis says. "If their patient feels that that their doctor is not interested in them as a person, but just as a hemoglobin A1C number, they find it really stressful."

The way that dynamic changes, Vallis believes, is when the patient and the doctor actually have an open and two-way conversation. "It's wonderful to have it at a presentation, but the way it's really going to change is when you sit down with Dr. Jones and say, 'Dr. Jones, why aren't you more interested in what my life experience is? Because I can't manage my disease without you actually understanding what my life is like.'"

Doctors want to help, but until the discussion shifts, it can be hard to make progress.

* * * * *

A bad experience with a health care provider was what put Halifax's Kylie Peacock's life in jeopardy and shaped how she managed her physical and mental health. Like many young people, Peacock faced a great deal of change when she moved from Ontario to attend Nova Scotia's Dalhousie University. Not only was she leaving her friends and family behind, but she also left the diabetes care team she'd been working with since she was first diagnosed with type 1 diabetes.

Peacock, who had an incident of extreme hypoglycemia as an undergrad, felt shamed and blamed by the resident who treated her. Already sensing she was out of place as a person with diabetes on a university campus, she was scared of burdening others with her fears. After the extreme low blood sugar event, she was determined to be more low-key about her diagnosis. So, she did what many people with type 1 do after an extreme low event—she kept her sugar levels intentionally high to avoid ever going low again. This strategy is as dangerous as it is common, as high blood sugar levels can cause long-term health complications.

"It wasn't until the end of my undergrad degree that I realized I needed to do something about this," Peacock says. She also had to start seeing a health care team again after dodging it for too long. "I think it really speaks to how even one interaction with a health care provider can really impact someone living with diabetes."

Peacock had dealt with mental health challenges in the past, including generalized anxiety disorder, so she decided to find a psychologist first. She hoped that getting her mental health sorted out would help her move on with the other issues she was managing. She spent some time online searching for a therapist who specialized in treating people with diabetes, and she eventually found Michael Vallis. She had no idea he was a leading expert on the topic, just that he was in Halifax, and if she went to the Dalhousie diabetes clinic and got a referral, he would see her. Suddenly, she not only had a psychologist who understood her diagnosis but had an entire health care team again.

"I thought that was very interesting because what I had not seen before was that there was a mental health care provider as part of the team. I didn't have to go seek my own psychologist," she says of the clinic's model of integrated care teams.

"The experience of meeting with a psychologist was a new one for me, and I was very nervous at first, but Michael has a way about him that makes you feel so comfortable. And some of the first words he said to me were, 'I understand how hard diabetes is, as well as chronic conditions and multiple morbidities.' For someone to just acknowledge that, as well as his depth of knowledge on chronic conditions and diabetes—the emotional impact was something I'd never heard before from any of my health care providers," she says.

"I've had diabetes now for almost 21 years, and 21 years ago we didn't have shared decision making or collaboration, so it was very paternalistic—'This is what I'm telling you to do.' And we did it," she says. "Health care providers can have such an impact on how you take care of yourself, whether it's a psychologist or an endocrinologist or a diabetes educator or diabetes nurse practitioner. Michael respected me and my story. When I told him that for years I'd kept my blood sugars high, there was this understanding that just made me so much more open to telling my story to him, and then to start telling my story to others." This relief is echoed by many who have finally seen a mental health expert who specializes in the disease.

It is common practice in therapy to ask a person to write down their fear and then to write down a balanced thought—something that shows how the fear is out of proportion with the reality. In diabetes, however, that is much more difficult. Someone who has an extreme fear of hypoglycemia has that fear because the condition can be terrifying and potentially fatal. Someone who fears developing complications like amputation or blindness has that fear legitimately because those are potential complications of diabetes. And so the cycle Peacock found herself in—keeping her sugars high in order to stave off hypoglycemia, and then having to manage the potential complications that arise from that—well, it's hard to find a balanced thought to reframe that.

For Vallis, who had long seen Peacock's behaviour in other patients with diabetes, her fear of hypoglycemia would not have come as a surprise. It's an area that, through the DAWN studies and his own research, he has come to realize is an enormous source of stress for those with the disease.

"Hypoglycemia is a fear problem before it is a glucose problem," he explains. "If your house is on fire and you have to jump out of a second-story window, you will do it, even though you know you might get hurt, but there is no choice because you have to escape. And you can't say to somebody, 'Well, just sit there, and maybe the fire department will come.' Because that's not human nature; we get out. Because it's a fear."

Avoidance, he says, is formed from that fear, as the person will do whatever they can to bypass that situation again. Suddenly, the calculation of what blood sugar range feels comfortable grows out of proportion. "If someone has a serious hypoglycemic episode, they usually increase that range because they think to themselves, 'What's that range where I know I won't go low? It used to be that I would leave my house, and I was OK if I was between 10 and 8, but now it's

14 and 12, because I know I can't go low if my sugars come down. And 15 is high, but 14 is acceptable.'"

This fear issue is not always an area well understood by other practitioners. And it's this desire by health care providers to simply treat the problem through direction—'You need to keep your sugars lower because it's important'—and not to address the underlying issues behind the decision to avoid hypoglycemia at all costs that becomes a vicious circle. Neither the doctor nor the patient feels heard, and the desired outcome does not happen.

At the 2019 Diabetes Canada Professional Conference, Adam Brown from diatTribe gave a keynote address. As a person living with diabetes, he has written much about the need to have an understanding of day-to-day life included in a person's treatment and care. His talk was in plain language, and it made good sense. He also offered simple, logical steps to help both patients and their care teams better integrate a person's life experience into their care plan.

Watching him, it was easy to see how much the DAWN studies had changed the way that health care providers were receiving this information. The room was packed, and the audience snapped dozens of photos of his slides, eager to consider how to put his words into their practice. For people with diabetes, this is a crucial moment in the progression of their care.

Vallis admits change is coming, though it is slow. "Inching, like a glacier moving," he says. "You ask a person living with diabetes, 'Have you ever felt judged by a health care provider? Do you ever feel like you're a kid being called into the principal's office? Do you ever feel like you're going to be scolded for what you didn't do? Do you ever feel this pressure to kind of lie, to tell the doctor or the educator what they want to hear?' Almost all of them will say they have.

"Even though in our heads we say intellectually, we believe that the psychological component is great, we still don't live it," he says. "I still think there needs to be a little bit of a shift in the attitude, which is what took my work in the direction of not only behaviour change in individuals living with disease but behaviour change in health care providers. What are the psychological changes around power, around complexity, around control that health care providers need to make in order to be better able to support the patient?"

For Vallis and others, the main goals are creating a collaborative, empowering, and caring relationship and supporting patients in completing the tasks in front of them.

Peacock is convinced this is crucial. Vallis is no longer her doctor since he left his position with the provincial health authority to pursue his research interests. His impact on her life is still a large one, however. It was during her work with him that she decided to pursue patient advocacy, realizing that by speaking out about her experience, she could help others. She now sits on numerous patient committees and is a frequent speaker at events.

"I feel like I'm at a point where I'm open to talk about my mental health and my diabetes," she says. "I think it depends on your goals, but I feel so great that I can go up on stage at a conference or speak with a research team about living with mental health issues and chronic conditions. I'm just one voice, but stories are so powerful. I've had some really unfortunate health care interactions, so how can we learn and do better? That's one thing Michael taught me so many years ago. Your voice can and should be included in these conversations. It shouldn't only be researchers in these conversations. Let them know what *you* want for your care."

CHAPTER TWELVE

The Ups and Downs of Diabetes and Exercise

Dessi Zaharieva seems tiny in person. Slender and fit, she stands only about 5'6" tall. She is quick to laugh and full of infectious energy and enthusiasm. In her blue blazer and grey slacks, her shoulder-length brown hair neatly styled, she looks very much like a graduate student about to defend her thesis, not a martial artist who goes by the nickname "The Bulgarian Bulldozer." In reality, she is both.

Zaharieva also has type 1 diabetes. Diagnosed at age seven, shortly after her family immigrated to Canada from Bulgaria, she has earned her reputation as a fighter. Having a child with type 1 diabetes is complicated. It involves learning a seemingly endless list of rules that must be followed in order to keep that child healthy and *alive*. For new immigrants who did not yet speak the language, it must have seemed an almost insurmountable situation.

Yet not only did the family manage, Zaharieva *thrived*. She is whip-smart and athletic. Her sport of choice, the martial arts, is not particularly well suited to a person with type 1 diabetes. But Zaharieva and her mentor—Dr. Michael Riddell, a professor in the department of kinesiology and health sciences at York University, as well as a world-leading expert on diabetes and exercise—strongly believe that someone with type 1 diabetes should be able to take part in whatever athletic pursuit they choose, whether it's basketball, skating, or combat sports.

Zaharieva's interest in martial arts started when she was young.

Shortly after her diagnosis, her father saw an ad in the paper for a Tae-kwondo class and enrolled her and her older brother. But any type of exercise is more complicated when you live with type 1 diabetes because you must constantly monitor blood sugars to ensure that levels do not spike or become dangerously low. For many with the disease, this can cause them to shy away from exercise, despite the positive impact it can have on their outcomes, but Zaharieva's parents refused to see it as a barrier.

"My family, we're not quitters, and we fight through everything as a family," Zaharieva tells me. Getting involved in a combat sport while managing a new and complicated diagnosis was a challenge, but she was determined, and her family was all in. Her brother, who is four years older, excelled in the sport, and his success inspired Zaharieva. "I was always competitive, from the time I was a kid," she says. "I wanted to reach his level, and he was just more talented than I was. I had a really hard time when I started because I actually wasn't very good at Taekwondo at all, but we're driven like that."

Zaharieva is not exaggerating when she talks about her drive. While she may have struggled in the sport initially, her tenacity kept her going back to practice every week, and she was soon fighting competitively. At the age of eighteen, she was the youngest member of the adult Taekwondo division for Team Canada. While her success at the sport was undeniable, her efforts to manage this level of competitive sport while living with diabetes were becoming more apparent.

"Low blood sugars are our biggest barrier to exercise," she says. "Hypoglycemia is the biggest fear. We don't want to be low while we're exercising—or overnight." Unfortunately, Zaharieva's blood sugar fluctuations led to several hospitalizations in her late teens, and they forced her to look closely at the realities of competing at this level of athletics with type 1 diabetes.

"I was really trying to understand what was going on with my diabetes, and a lot of it had to do with trying to cut body weight for competition, compete at the highest level, follow a very strict diet, and make weight. It was just a lot all at the same time, and not knowing enough about exercise and diabetes because there was nothing available at the time," she says. "The hospitalizations didn't happen just because I wasn't taking care of myself properly. A lot of it happened because of post-exercise hypoglycemia overnight. We go to sleep, and our blood sugars go low, and I just didn't know enough about that."

These days, people with type 1 diabetes have access to many technology-based solutions, and an insulin pump and continuous glucose monitor (CGM) have made an enormous difference for Zaharieva and other type 1 athletes. CGM does exactly what the name implies—it attaches to the body and provides ongoing updates to blood sugar levels, alerting the wearer of any fluctuations in order to help keep glucose levels stable.

An insulin pump is also worn on the body and ensures that blood glucose levels don't go too high or too low, giving low doses of insulin throughout the day and allowing the wearer to increase the amount of insulin if needed. For many people, it's a better and more seamless option than injections, but it involves a lot of maintenance. And wearing it can be cumbersome, especially when you're taking part in sports.

Zaharieva can't fight with her pump on, nor can she train. The pump could be kicked off or ripped from her body in a fight, so it's simply not realistic to wear it. But after just an hour without it, her blood sugars can start to fluctuate significantly, and without the CGM to alert her, she's at a disadvantage.

"Your doctor always says, 'Don't take it off for more than an hour.' Well, my training sessions are sometimes two hours, sometimes three hours, and I reconnect my pump usually right at the end of training. Then I have to take a small dose of insulin to try and correct for the amount of insulin that I missed, sooner rather than later," Zaharieva explains. "The struggle is that the action of insulin is still so slow. We talk about all these fast insulins, and none of them are really as fast as they should be or could be. That would be the best thing for myself and for all people living with diabetes. If we can get that insulin into the circulation faster, it would just make it a lot easier to manage our condition."

On fight days, when stress can cause unusual fluctuations in blood sugar, Zaharieva turns to visualizations and other meditative techniques to calm her nerves and keep her blood sugars as stable as possible. Unless she's already running high, she keeps her pump on until just before a match and puts it on as soon as she can afterwards. It's not perfect, but it's far better now, in her late twenties, than it was in her teenage years.

The changes she has made are in part due to the scientific research projects she herself has worked on. When Zaharieva realized there weren't enough answers to the questions she had about how to compete as a top-level athlete with type 1 diabetes, she decided to start trying to uncover them herself. This is what led her to Dr. Michael Riddell's lab at York University.

* * * * *

Dr. Michael Riddell walks into a tiny research lab at LMC Healthcare and immediately starts to chat with the woman whose blood is being taken. He introduces himself, asks how she's feeling, exchanges a bit of chitchat about the study she's taking part in—then he spots her insulin pump. Immediately, he's curious, asking questions about what he quickly recognizes as newly approved technology in Canada. He knows that she would have had to get hers in the U.S. The patient beams, thrilled to show off the top-of-the-line insulin pump.

They discuss how much insulin the sleek machine can hold given its relatively small size (it's smaller than the average cell phone) and how it can be updated like a smartphone when there are upgrades to the software, a huge step up from the current situation, where those on a pump must often wait years to purchase the newer model and get the latest upgrades.

Heather Worboys is blonde, pretty, middle-aged, and very fit. A nurse, she has lived with type 1 diabetes since 1996, and she's happy to lend her time to research like Riddell's, which can help improve her glucose control during exercise. Now she talks animatedly about how the pump is improving her glucose management.

Riddell notes that his research assistant, Sarah, who is stationed behind him, watching over the process of blood being drawn, is hoping to get this type of model once her insurance will cover an upgrade. Worboys nods in understanding. These are the sort of issues that come up a lot when you're using technology to manage a chronic disease; it can be challenging to wait for the latest upgrade. Almost everyone in this small, crowded room seems to have type 1 diabetes, save for the technicians currently managing the blood draw—and me. In the moments since we entered the room, it is clear that Riddell, who arguably has the most knowledge of any of us, has endless questions for those around him.

I have seen Riddell in these types of conversations several times over the years. He listens intently, asks questions, and offers suggestions. I waited for him once after a presentation he gave at Diabetes Canada's Type 1 Conference. A long line had formed, as more than a dozen people who had just watched him speak waited patiently for their turn to ask him questions. They would make their way to him, tell him how long they'd had diabetes, the sport they played or the exercise they did, and explain the results they were seeing in their blood sugars. Riddell considered each question, asked about their pumps or CGM, and offered suggestions and ideas.

He laughs easily and exudes a warmth that draws people to him like a magnet. As I continued waiting for him, admittedly a bit impatiently by the end as we ticked further and further off schedule, it was fascinating to watch. It was as if one of the busiest researchers in the country had all the time in the world for people living with diabetes. And in many ways, he does.

Riddell was diagnosed with type 1 diabetes at age fourteen. His diagnosis left him shaken and overwhelmed, but it also became the catalyst for his career. "I think it defines me," he says of how the disease has shaped the work to which he's dedicated his life. "I think it defines every research study I do, every grant I write, every manuscript I read. It's just always with me."

In Angela Duckworth's book, *Grit: The Power of Passion and Perseverance*, she discusses how research has shown that hard work often trumps natural talent—that it is those who struggle with something initially, but who are determined to master it anyway, who may achieve the highest level of success. I thought of Riddell often as I read her book. A self-described average student, it was Riddell's diabetes diagnosis and his determination to remain a competitive athlete that drove him to learn everything he could about how to overcome this challenge. He is, without question, someone with an incredible amount of grit.

In his presentations, Riddell often speaks about how his ambitions changed drastically after his diagnosis. He went from having no interest in pursuing a career in science or academia to studying kinesiology and developing a deep fascination with how the body works, and the role type 1 diabetes played in pursuing his athletic goals. Sports were an important part of his life, and he wanted to know how to manage his blood sugars to compete at his maximum potential. He also wanted to help others do the same.

"Something about that diagnosis put me on the right path," he says. "I was interested in exercise. I was pretty active as a teenager and fascinated by metabolism, like why is it your body responds differently to different forms of exercise? I started to study pretty hard after my diagnosis, and eventually, I decided I wanted to do a PhD in the area."

Riddell attended McMaster University in Hamilton, Ontario, studying under the late Dr. Oded Bar-Or, who founded the Children's Exercise and Nutrition Centre at McMaster Children's Hospital in 1983. It was under Bar-Or's tutelage that Riddell began to look into type 1 diabetes and exercise. From there, he found a mentor in Dr. Mladen Vranic, a legendary figure in diabetes research, who in 1963, had been invited to work in Canada by Dr. Charles Best, the co-discoverer of insulin.

Vranic, who passed away in 2019, is credited with some of the world's most influential research on exercise and diabetes—in particular, in the area of using exercise to prevent or lessen the impact of type 2 diabetes. His mentorship helped Riddell narrow his research focus. While Vranic had done much to move forward the scientific understanding of type 2 diabetes and exercise, Riddell realized how little was understood about type 1 diabetes and competitive sport.

"Working with Mladen was one of the most important opportunities I have had professionally," Riddell says of the role his mentor played in helping define his career path. "Mladen had always been fascinated by how exercise and stress influence diabetes-related metabolism. He is recognized as one of the leaders in the field of diabetes and metabolism, and he taught me to use my own experiences with diabetes to influence the research questions that I ask. He felt that living with type 1 diabetes would offer me lots of opportunities in life, both personally and professionally, and it has."

Tall and athletic, Riddell continued to play basketball and cycle. He was passionate about sport and frustrated by the idea that having type 1 diabetes could potentially limit his abilities. The lack of research into this subject concerned him. He wanted to understand why sometimes a competitive match shot his blood sugars up and why other times he went low. There were so few studies that looked at athletic pursuits at a level beyond the average.

There are many professional athletes who live with type 1 diabetes, so why was there so little research being done about it?

Riddell's wife, Sara, a sports executive, shares his passion for athletics. She is also the daughter of a woman with type 1 diabetes, giving her an understanding of the condition that deeply mattered to Riddell. When he speaks about his wife, his face lights up, as it does when he talks about their three children. Sara's relationship with the disease, however, has come with risks.

The genetic link to type 1 diabetes is complicated and not entirely understood. Anecdotally, as someone who works with people living with the disease, I can tell you it's not uncommon to see it run in families. Given that Riddell and his mother-in-law live with type 1, all three of his children needed to be monitored closely for the condition. Riddell did not primarily focus on this, however. He started his research program, developed a reputation as one of the best in his field, and began working with the DSkate program to help get kids with type 1 diabetes involved in hockey. He built a career and a life where his three kids grew up surrounded by a community of those living with type 1 diabetes. All around them, people tested their blood sugars, counted carbs, and talked about insulin, test strips, and CGM.

You can never be truly prepared when your child is diagnosed with a chronic illness—one they will live with for the rest of their life, especially one you yourself have lived with for almost forty years. When Riddell tells the story of his oldest son Sam's diagnosis, he talks about how, even knowing the risks, even understanding diabetes so well, it completely knocked the wind out of him.

He speaks with awe about how Sam, a thirteen-year-old who had grown up surrounded by type 1 diabetes, gave himself his first-ever injection. He'd watched it done so many times that he needed no instruction. The medical staff had never seen anything like it.

Today, chatting with the research subject in his lab, Riddell tells her that his son would probably like her new pump. "Your son has diabetes, too?" she asks, a look of surprise flashing across her face. "Yep," Riddell replies as if it's the most normal thing in the world. Sam's diagnosis may have been a blow, but it has made Riddell even more dedicated to this work.

"I didn't realize that being a parent would really change my perspective on the research that needs to be done—and more than the research—the education and the support that needs to be done," he says. "If we invent all these tools and technologies, but we don't get adolescents to use them or appreciate them, then it's a waste of time and energy because we have to support these kids as they mature with their diabetes."

This new perspective has shaped his thinking about what people with diabetes actually need to be successful in sport and in life. He considers not just his own experiences but what is different about how his son manages his diabetes compared with how he managed his own as a young adult. It has also made Riddell think hard about how research is made relatable outside the lab—how were doctors and scientists talking to children and teens—and to their parents—about these issues? "Now I think the projects we do outside our research, like DSkate Hockey and the York Diabetes Sports Camp, and all the events where we get together with other parents or kids, are probably more important than any of the research I do."

At DSkate, where kids are encouraged to learn to self-manage their diabetes while participating in a sport they enjoy, the team provides a fun and active environment, as well as educational seminars about diabetes management and technologies. "Most of them come away from that camp with more confidence around diabetes, and more willingness to try technology and to take ownership of their disease, rather than leave it up to their parents or just ignore it altogether," he says of the program.

"I am always exhausted when I'm done those camps, and I always think going into them, 'Do I have the energy to do this *and* maintain a lab *and* be a parent and a husband *and* travel all over the world?' And then those weeks are just invigorating for me because I see all the gaps and the problems, so it informs me for the next twelve months."

The camps and programs bring the reality of life with diabetes into stark focus for Riddell, and spending time with these kids is inspiring and enlightening. Having had the opportunity to visit Diabetes Canada's D-Camps program, which provides children with diabetes a traditional summer camp experience in a medically-supervised environment, I understand the impact this interaction can have. People often think only of the limiting factors of a life with type 1 diabetes, but seeing healthy, happy kids engaged in fun activities, counting carbs and taking injections, yes, but *also* laughing and singing and being kids, makes you want to figure out ways to ensure that their lives can be just as full at all times.

Like Riddell, I was blown away by the talents and athletic acumen of the kids I met at the D-Camps program, and it helped me gain a stronger understanding of Riddell's motivation. And after my rather disastrous attempt at archery, I also realize how the usually very athletic Riddell must feel whenever he runs a hockey camp, and the kids realize he's incredibly inept on ice skates.

It is these real-life interactions that inspired Riddell's recent work on an exercise-management app for people with diabetes. One of the most unique aspects of diabetes is that it *is* unique. What you eat, how much you exercise, the stress you are under, and even your sleep patterns can all have an impact on your blood glucose. This is why experts in the area will tell you there is not a one-size-fits-all solution to living with the condition. Riddell's exercise planner takes these things into consideration and is based on the Canadian and international exercise and type 1 diabetes guidelines he has helped to develop. In many cases, he has been the lead on these projects.

The main idea is to take what is known about diabetes and exercise and build that into the app. The user can then determine their goals, be they weight loss or performance improvements, input their specific information, and receive data reports that show their progress and support their goals. The information is also available for their health care teams to ensure they are working together to successfully support the person's health.

The app, which Riddell is working on with a large life sciences firm, is awaiting FDA approval when we talk, but he's hopeful it will pass. He sees this type of technology as a next step for those trying to manage their diabetes and exercise goals as the field transitions to better support young people in ways that will work for them.

He has also started looking deeply into how exercise can be studied outside a lab environment. In science, controls are important. You want people to do the exact same things at the exact same times under the exact same conditions and having eaten (or more frequently, *not* eaten) the exact same things. Studies done under these conditions are extremely valuable to moving forward our understanding of physiological responses. But life is not like that.

As wearable technologies like insulin pumps and CGM develop, it is allowing Riddell to better study people "in the wild" and to look for solutions that will speak to their specific needs. "Most of us exercise with varying amounts of food and bolus insulin in our bodies, so the research landscape is now trying to include more real-life scenarios," he explains, noting that his lab and others in the field are doing more large data studies outside of the clinic now that these devices give them tools to measure results in a way that didn't exist before.

He is also continuing the work he started with Vranic, looking for ways to prevent hypoglycemia during exercise. When Vranic retired, Riddell took over the projects that were showing the most promise, and one has since spun out into a start-up company called Zucara Therapeutics.

When someone with diabetes experiences an extreme low, glucagon is needed to reverse that effect. Currently, there is no way to regulate this easily, but Riddell's work looks at injecting a hormone or taking a drug that affects the glucagon-producing alpha cells so that when someone goes low, the body produces the needed glucagon response. If it works, Riddell explains, the drug has the promise of cutting hypoglycemia substantially.

He has also been looking at the potential benefits of injecting glucagon into people before they exercise. "You can take a little bit of soluble glucagon and inject it five minutes before you exercise, and your blood sugar stays flat. So that's kind of exciting," he says.

Talking about these projects, an app to customize your exercise management, a drug to prevent hypoglycemia during your workout, an injection that keeps your blood sugars flat, Riddell's enthusiasm is clear. He is also realistic, however, in particular around drug-related therapies. "I want to be the person who is known for having developed a library of tools to make exercise safer and more accessible for diabetes, whether it's a new drug or a new therapeutic approach or a new style of exercise. That's my passion," he says. "But if we develop a drug that is a whole new class of medication to prevent hypoglycemia, the first new medication for type 1 since insulin was discovered, that would be massive. But that's a team approach that has high risk."

Such is the way for all scientists—your goal is to fix something without breaking something else. For people who live with the disease they aim to treat, this is perhaps even more critical. The stakes are much higher when you are working on something that may change your own life or that of your child.

* * * * *

That Dessi Zaharieva ended up working with Michael Riddell should come as no surprise. When you meet them, it's immediately clear they both possess the same courage and determination needed to succeed in the type of athleticism and research that drives them.

Yet Zaharieva tells me Riddell was not entirely certain about taking on his first trainee with type 1 diabetes. She had completed her undergraduate studies in kinesiology and was trying to decide where to go from there. She had considered studying thermoregulation, but something kept tugging her back towards type 1 and exercise.

"At that time, I was competing for Team Canada, but for the adult category, so now there was even more pressure," she tells me. "You're not really considered a junior anymore; you're kind of stepping into the real world. I was the youngest athlete on Team Canada because it goes from age eighteen to thirty-nine for adults. So I have this whole new ballpark where I have to succeed in sport but also understand my diabetes. I looked up researchers online who do type 1 diabetes and exercise-related research, and Dr. Riddell came up."

Zaharieva reached out, and she and Riddell began the interview process. It was clear she had the potential to be an excellent scientist and had the needed qualifications, but Riddell was hesitant.

"I remember when we met telling him that I have type 1, and he said, 'It's not about your capabilities or what you can do as a researcher or as a person. I just worry that being immersed in diabetes research all the time, you're teaching, you're educating, you're learning about it. And then you remove yourself from that, and you're living it, you're breathing it, you're sleeping it, you're thinking about it all the time. You don't really have a moment to shut off from it.' I think I was his first student ever with type 1 diabetes because he knew how challenging that could be, even for me. A lot of people get diabetes without being immersed in this as a job, and it was really nice that he thought about that and made me aware of it."

The warning did not deter Zaharieva, nor the other trainees with diabetes who have since joined Riddell's lab. He admits that he sometimes still worries about this in his own life, especially now that he is also the parent of a child with type 1 diabetes. Is it too much to live and breathe and work in type 1 diabetes? For researchers like Zaharieva and himself, they cannot imagine having it any other way.

For Riddell's part, he now sees Zaharieva as the future of this work. "She's going to be the replacement for me when I finally want to retire from this field if I ever do," he says with a chuckle, though he's completely serious.

Having earned her doctorate in 2018, Zaharieva is following her passion and continuing to study technological advancements in type 1 diabetes, specifically around exercise. She is fascinated with closed-loop systems and the artificial pancreas. In Riddell's lab, they have studied the response of CGM and other technologies during intensive exercise—and have grown concerned that the systems don't always respond accurately under these conditions.

This fact is not entirely surprising, given that the devices were developed and tested using patients who were performing fairly standard activities. At rest, the devices are highly accurate, but when a person is playing competitive sports, there is often a lag in giving accurate blood glucose levels. For an athlete with diabetes, this is a major concern. "We know that one of the biggest challenges right now is getting these systems working well during exercise," says Zaharieva. "We have to remember that these are just systems at the end of the day, so there's a lot that needs to be integrated into them to improve their accuracy."

As these devices become more common and increasingly available for people with type 1 diabetes, Zaharieva sees her role moving forward as helping to ensure they are safe and effective for athletes. While she may never be able to wear a pump in a martial arts match, as the devices get smaller and more precise there may come a time when her research helps to make that possible. Or Riddell's glucagon therapy may remove the need for pumps during sport altogether.

The results of their research projects, like all science, is unknowable, but their work continues to lead the path forward to improved treatments. Riddell is immensely proud of the work his protégé is doing, and while his initial concerns about her being so immersed in diabetes were valid, he has realized what those of us looking in from the outside knew long ago: Despite the incredible contributions of other scientists in the field, it is the person with type 1 diabetes, who understands what it's like to smack into the barriers presented by their body, who is the person most likely to figure out how to smash through them.

The "Bulgarian Bulldozer" seems primed for this challenge.

Afterword
Priye Iworima, MSc

When Krista approached me about writing the afterword for her book, I was excited and honoured. While we have much to be grateful for from Banting and the many talented researchers who have continued to work towards improved treatments and cures, the future is full of even more promise.

In my own work, I've always been fascinated by mysteries and problem-solving. This curiosity led me down the not-so-straightforward path to where I am today: working with stem cells in a lab at the University of British Columbia to make insulin-producing cells. It is a journey that excites me because it has introduced me to a group of people working towards the common goal of trying to find a cure for diabetes. This journey has immersed me in a community of amazing people who walk together, grow with each other, challenge each other, and uplift each other.

Science is done by people and for people. Those living with diabetes inspire me, and they shape research questions and outcomes. They are the reason so many scientists feel compelled to do this work. Because of numerous research and funding agencies, I've had the pleasure to meet and interact with many beautiful people living with diabetes. They have graciously shared their stories of triumph and successes, as well as the challenges they face daily, either in efforts to manage their diabetes or deal with the stigma and discrimination they often encounter.

I recently received a letter from Alan, who has lived with type 1 diabetes for 53 years. He recounted the ups and downs he has faced since his diagnosis. He also talked about his excitement for the research we're doing and how it has the potential to change millions of lives. I am amazed at the grit, and fortitude people have. And every time I get to hear an impact statement from participants in a clinical trial, it only makes me strive harder to contribute in some way towards the goal of finding a cure for diabetes.

This book tells the story of research teams across Canada who are working hard to make a difference in the lives of people living with diabetes. I feel lucky to work and learn from many of them and to have the chance to be part of a collaborative and supportive community. I also feel inspired by the students and future scientists who will shape this sector in the future. We won't stop until we find a cure.

We live in interesting times, where looking a certain way is often the sole basis for judgment and for people defining you and your abilities. Don't ever let that quench your shine! You can do and be whatever you set your mind to be. To that little girl dreaming of becoming a scientist, to that little Black boy wondering what the future holds and how society has defined you, and to everyone who feels out of place in the world simply because you are "different," remember that the future looks like you and me. When the road gets rough, surround yourself with an amazing support system. You are not in this alone, and I can't wait to see how you continue to make this world a better place.

Acknowledgements

It takes a village to write a book—in particular, a book like this where I interviewed dozens of people and was supported by a group of family, friends and colleagues who went above and beyond to help make this project a reality. I am incredibly grateful.

My dad, Donald, passed away in 2007. Leading up to his death, we talked a lot about my future, and he reminded me yet again that he hoped one day I'd write a book. Seeing this project come to fruition, I often think of his love and support and how that drove me on the days when I thought this project was just too big.

My mom, Colleen, has been a tireless supporter. She never doubted that I could do this and never stopped telling me how proud of me she was.

My husband, Shawn, has been a constant source of encouragement. Every time I hit a roadblock, he was there to help me plow through it. That kind of love can move mountains—or get a book published.

I was out with a group of girlfriends in 2018 when I first expressed the idea for this project out loud. Maybe it was the wine or the warmth of that circle of friends, but their enthusiasm that night lit the spark that gave this project life. They have continued to encourage me along the way: Kim, Amanda and Natalie, thanks for telling me I could do this.

My editor, Tara Mandarano, is one of the best writers I know. She is also a fantastic editor. And a tireless advocate and friend. I'm so glad we got to do this together.

The mentors in my life have been both inspirations and friends. Each has taken a chance on me, and in doing so, allowed me to grow as a writer, a communicator, and a human: Anya Wilson, Lisa McKeen, Jan Hux, and Bruce Perkins—thank you.

An enormous thanks to David Hayes, who guided me as a journalism student and then took me seriously when I invited him out for breakfast and said, "I have this idea..." Your support and advice throughout this process have been invaluable.

Jodi Garner took the time to read each of these chapters to help check the science. She also listened to me talk endlessly about this project, and she didn't murder me. She's a good friend.

Zoë Gemelli took my author photos and helped with the final edit of the book—thanks for making me look so good!

There were a lot of days where I didn't think I'd be able to make it through so many things—Nik Grujich made sure I always did. He also listened to me talk endlessly about terrible novels that never made it past my computer screen. This book truly wouldn't be possible without him.

A huge thank you to the kind friends who let me spend a summer as their unofficial writer in residence, allowing me to actually finish this book on time during the months of unending construction in my usual writing space. You will never appreciate silence more than when you have tried to start a business, finish a book and record a podcast series while people sand concrete outside your door.

When the book was nearing completion, and I needed people to help fact check, I was amazed at how, in the middle of a global pandemic that had upended many of their lives and careers, so many of Canada's diabetes research community said yes when I asked for a favour. Enormous thanks to Drs. Jenny Bruin, Alice Cheng, David Campbell, Jan Hux, James Johnson, Lorraine Lipscombe, Erin Mulvihill, Bruce Perkins, Michael Riddell, and Peter Senior for stepping up to assist with this.

It was the *Diabetes Canada Podcast* that inspired me to write this book, and I am grateful to the team at Diabetes Canada for allowing me to use content from those interviews within these pages. Thanks, in particular to the wonderful editors I have worked with there, Teigan Reamsbottom and Raquel Dominguez. I am also grateful to all those who have listened and spread the word about this project.

In addition, I have had the support of an incredible group of friends and colleagues over the last three years who have leant an ear, read a draft, or listened to yet another research story: Amy, Hanna, Suzie, Eva, Ryan L., Ryan M, Elesha, Angela, Donna, Catriona, Megan, Charlene, Krista B., Kari, Paul D., Marc, Stella, Paul K., Matt, Lena, Grace, Denise, Pilar, Hillary, Stephanie, Tracy, Meg, and all the others I may have missed. You were all part of making this book a reality.

There were many stories I didn't get to tell in these pages. I hope to have the opportunity to tell them in other ways. If you are interested in this work or the work of other scientists in Canada, please visit my website at kristalamb.com to see more of my writing.

Recommended Reading

The Sisterhood of Diabetes: Facing Challenges & Living Dreams by Judith Ambrosini

The Discovery of Insulin by Michael Bliss

Bright Spots & Landmines: The Diabetes Guide I Wish Someone had Handed Me by Adam Brown

Grit by Angela Duckworth

The Diet Fix: Why Diets Fail and How to Make Yours Work by Yoni Freedhoff

Diagnosing the Legacy: The Discovery, Research, and Treatment of Type 2 Diabetes in Indigenous Youth by Larry Krotz

Ask Me About My Uterus: A Quest to Make Doctors Believe in Women's Pain by Abby Norman

Getting Pumped: An Insulin Pump Guide for Active Individuals with Type 1 Diabetes by Michael Riddell

Dreams and Due Diligence: Till and McCulloch's Stem Cell Discovery and Legacy by Joe Sornberger

Recommended Listening

Actions on Diabetes Podcast
From Beta cells to Bicycles Podcast
Diabetes Canada Podcast
Missed in History Class: The Discovery of Insulin, Parts 1 and 2
Stem Cell Podcast

Selected References

Chapter One

Canadian Agency for Drugs and Technologies in Health Care (CADTH) Health Economics Working Group, CADTH Guidelines for the Economic Evaluation of Health Technologies, 4th edition, 2017.

Drucker DJ. The Ascending GLP-1 Road From Clinical Safety to Reduction of Cardiovascular Complications. *Diabetes.* 2018;67(9):1710-1719. doi:10.2337/dbi18-0008.

Drucker DJ, Habener JF, Holst JJ. Discovery, characterization, and clinical development of the glucagon-like peptides. *J Clin Invest.* 2017;127(12):4217-4227. doi:10.1172/JCI97233.

Drucker DJ, Nauck MA. The incretin system: glucagon-like peptide-1 receptor agonists and dipeptidyl peptidase-4 inhibitors in type 2 diabetes. Lancet. 2006 Nov 11;368(9548):1696-705. doi: 10.1016/S0140-6736(06)69705-5. PMID: 17098089.

Baggio LL, Drucker DJ. Biology of incretins: GLP-1 and GIP. Gastroenterology. 2007 May;132(6):2131-57. doi: 10.1053/j.gastro.2007.03.054. PMID: 17498508.

Drucker DJ. The biology of incretin hormones. Cell Metab. 2006 Mar;3(3):153-65. doi: 10.1016/j.cmet.2006.01.004. PMID: 16517403.

Chapter Two

Agarwal P, Morriseau TS, Kereliuk SM, Doucette CA, Wicklow BA, Dolinsky VW. Maternal obesity, diabetes during pregnancy and epigenetic mechanisms that influence the developmental origins of cardiometabolic disease in the offspring. Crit Rev Clin Lab Sci. 2018 Mar;55(2):71-101. doi: 10.1080/10408363.2017.1422109. Epub 2018 Jan 8. PMID: 29308692.

Dart AB, Wicklow B, Blydt-Hansen TD, Sellers EAC, Malik S, Chateau D, Sharma A, McGavock JM. A Holistic Approach to Risk for Early Kidney Injury in Indigenous Youth With Type 2 Diabetes: A Proof of Concept Paper From the iCARE Cohort. Can J Kidney Health Dis. 2019 Apr 21;6:2054358119838836. doi: 10.1177/2054358119838836. PMID: 31041107; PMCID: PMC6477761.

Dart AB, Wicklow BA, Sellers EA, Dean HJ, Malik S, Walker J, Chateau D, Blydt-Hansen TD, McGavock JM; iCARE investigators. The Improving Renal Complications in Adolescents With Type 2 Diabetes Through the REsearch (iCARE) Cohort Study: rationale and Protocol. Can J Diabetes. 2014 Oct;38(5):349-55. doi: 10.1016/j.jcjd.2014.07.224. PMID: 25284698.

Dean HJ, Mundy RL, Moffatt M. Non-insulin-dependent diabetes mellitus in Indian children in Manitoba. CMAJ. 1992 Jul 1;147(1):52-7. PMID: 1393888; PMCID: PMC1336119.

Young TK, Martens PJ, Taback SP, Sellers EA, Dean HJ, Cheang M, Flett B. Type 2 diabetes mellitus in children: prenatal and early infancy risk factors among native Canadians. Arch Pediatr Adolesc Med. 2002 Jul;156(7):651-5. doi: 10.1001/archpedi.156.7.651. PMID: 12090830.

Dean H. NIDDM-Y in First Nation children in Canada. Clin Pediatr (Phila). 1998 Feb;37(2):89-96. doi: 10.1177/000992289803700205. PMID: 9492116.

Dean H. Diagnostic criteria for non-insulin dependent diabetes in youth (NIDDM-Y). Clin Pediatr (Phila). 1998 Feb;37(2):67-71. doi: 10.1177/000992289803700202. PMID: 9492113.

Jonasson ME, Wicklow BA, Sellers EA, Dolinsky VW, Doucette CA. Exploring the role of the HNF-1αG319S polymorphism in β cell failure and youth-onset type 2 diabetes: Lessons from MODY and Hnf-1α-deficient animal models. Biochem Cell Biol. 2015 Oct;93(5):487-94. doi-10.1139/bcb-2015-0021. Epub 2015 May 6. PMID: 26176428.

Maple-Brown LJ, Graham S, McKee J, Wicklow B. Walking the path together: incorporating Indigenous knowledge in diabetes research. Lancet Diabetes Endocrinol. 2020 Jul;8(7):559-560. doi: 10.1016/S2213-8587(20)30188-1. PMID: 32559468.

McGavock J, Sellers E, Dean H. Physical activity for the prevention and management of youth-onset type 2 diabetes mellitus: focus on cardiovascular complications. Diab Vasc Dis Res. 2007 Dec;4(4):305-10. doi: 10.3132/dvdr.2007.057. PMID: 18158700.

McGavock, J, Wicklow, B, Dart, Allison. Type 2 diabetes in youth is a disease of poverty. The Lancet. 2017, Oct. 21.

McGavock J, Dart A, Wicklow B. Lifestyle therapy for the treatment of youth with type 2 diabetes. Curr Diab Rep. 2015 Jan;15(1):568. doi: 10.1007/s11892-014-0568-z. PMID: 25398207; PMCID: PMC4232742.

Morriseau TS, Wicklow BA, Lavallee B. Intergenerational Impacts of Colonization: Outcomes of Diabetes in Pregnancy for First Nations Families. Can J Diabetes. 2020 Oct;44(7):573-574. doi: 10.1016/j.jcjd.2020.08.099. PMID: 32972639.

Sawatsky L, Halipchuk J, Wicklow B. Type 2 diabetes in a four-year-old child. CMAJ. 2017 Jul 4;189(26):E888-E890. doi: 10.1503/cmaj.170259. PMID: 28676579; PMCID: PMC5495639.

Sellers EA, Triggs-Raine B, Rockman-Greenberg C, Dean HJ. The prevalence of the HNF-1alpha G319S mutation in Canadian aboriginal youth with type 2 diabetes. Diabetes Care. 2002 Dec;25(12):2202-6. doi: 10.2337/diacare.25.12.2202. PMID: 12453961.

Wicklow BA, Sellers EA. Maternal health issues and cardio-metabolic outcomes in the offspring: a focus on Indigenous populations. Best Pract Res Clin Obstet Gynaecol. 2015 Jan;29(1):43-53. doi: 10.1016/j.bpobgyn.2014.04.017. Epub 2014 Aug 20. PMID: 25238683.

Wicklow BA, Sellers EAC, Sharma AK, Kroeker K, Nickel NC, Philips-Beck W, Shen GX. Association of Gestational Diabetes and Type 2 Diabetes Exposure In Utero With the Development of Type 2 Diabetes in First Nations and Non-First Nations Offspring. JAMA Pediatr. 2018 Aug 1;172(8):724-731. doi: 10.1001/jamapediatrics.2018.1201. PMID: 29889938; PMCID: PMC6142931.

Chapter Three

Ahmed A, Bril V, Orszag A, Paulson J, Yeung E, Ngo M, Orlov S, Perkins BA. Detection of diabetic sensorimotor polyneuropathy by corneal confocal microscopy in type 1 diabetes: a concurrent validity study. Diabetes Care. 2012 Apr 1;35(4):821-8.

Bril V, Perkins BA. Validation of the Toronto Clinical Scoring System for diabetic polyneuropathy. *Diabetes Care.* 2002;25(11):2048-2052. doi:10.2337/diacare.25.11.2048.

Diabetes Control and Complications Trial Research Group, Nathan DM, Genuth S, Lachin J, Cleary P, Crofford O, Davis M, Rand L, Siebert C. The effect of intensive treatment of diabetes on the development and progression of long-term complications in insulin-dependent diabetes mellitus. N Engl J Med. 1993 Sep 30;329(14):977-86. doi: 10.1056/NEJM199309303291401. PMID: 8366922.

Heerspink HJ, Perkins BA, Fitchett DH, Husain M, Cherney DZ. Sodium Glucose Cotransporter 2 Inhibitors in the Treatment of Diabetes Mellitus: Cardiovascular and Kidney Effects, Potential Mechanisms, and Clinical Applications. Circulation. 2016 Sep 6;134(10):752-72. doi: 10.1161/CIRCULATIONAHA.116.021887. Epub 2016 Jul 28. PMID: 27470878.

Del Degan S, Dubé F, Gagnon C, Boulet G. Risk Factors for Recurrent Diabetic Ketoacidosis in Adults With Type 1 Diabetes. Can J Diabetes. 2019 Oct;43(7):472-476.e1. doi: 10.1016/j.jcjd.2019.01.008. Epub 2019 Jan 28. PMID: 30853268.

Mohajeri S, Perkins BA, Brubaker PL, Riddell MC. Diabetes, trekking and high altitude: recognizing and preparing for the risks. Diabet Med. 2015 Nov;32(11):1425-37. doi: 10.1111/dme.12795. Epub 2015 May 30. PMID: 25962798.

Perkins BA, Olaleye D, Zinman B, Bril V. Simple screening tests for peripheral neuropathy in the diabetes clinic. *Diabetes Care.* 2001;24(2):250-256. doi:10.2337/diacare.24.2.250.

Perkins BA, Ficociello LH, Silva KH, Finkelstein DM, Warram JH, Krolewski AS. Regression of microalbuminuria in type 1 diabetes. *N Engl J Med.* 2003;348(23):2285-2293. doi:10.1056/NEJMoa021835.

Perkins BA, Bril V. Diabetic neuropathy: a review emphasizing diagnostic methods. *Clin Neurophysiol.* 2003;114(7):1167-1175. doi:10.1016/s1388-2457(03)00025-7.

Perkins BA, Cherney DZ, Partridge H, Soleymanlou N, Tschirhart H, Zinman B, Fagan NM, Kaspers S, Woerle HJ, Broedl UC, Johansen OE. Sodium-glucose cotransporter 2 inhibition and glycemic control in type 1 diabetes: results of an 8-week open-label proof-of-concept trial. Diabetes Care. 2014 May 1;37(5):1480-3.

Perkins BA, Lovblom LE, Bril V, Scarr D, Ostrovski I, Orszag A, Edwards K, Pritchard N, Russell A, Dehghani C, Pacaud D, Romanchuk K, Mah JK, Jeziorska M, Marshall A, Shtein RM, Pop-Busui R, Lentz SI, Boulton AJM, Tavakoli M, Efron N, Malik RA. Corneal confocal microscopy for identification of diabetic sensorimotor polyneuropathy: a pooled multinational consortium study. Diabetologia. 2018 Aug 1;61(8):1856-1861. 29869146.

Perkins BA, Rosenstock J, Skyler JS, Laffel LM, Cherney DZ, Mathieu C, Pang C, Wood R, Kinduryte O, George JT, Marquard J, Soleymanlou N. Exploring Patient Preferences for Adjunct-to-Insulin Therapy in Type 1 Diabetes. Diabetes

Care. 2019 Sep;42(9):1716-1723. doi: 10.2337/dc19-0548. Epub 2019 Jun 8. PMID: 31177179; PMCID: PMC6973543.

Perkins BA, Soleymanlou N, Rosenstock J, Skyler JS, Laffel LM, Liesenfeld KH, Neubacher D, Riggs MM, Johnston CK, Eudy-Byrne RJ, Elmokadem A, George JT, Marquard J, Nock V. Low-Dose Empagliflozin as Adjunct-to-Insulin Therapy in Type 1 Diabetes: A Valid Modeling and Simulation Analysis to Confirm Efficacy. Diabetes Obes Metab. 2019 Dec 19.

Rosenstock J, Marquard J, Laffel LM, Neubacher D, Kaspers S, Cherney DZ, Zinman B, Skyler JS, George J, Soleymanlou N, Perkins BA. Empagliflozin as Adjunctive to Insulin Therapy in Type 1 Diabetes: The EASE Trials. Diabetes Care. 2018 Dec 1;41(12):2560-2569. 30287422.

Sivaskandarajah GA, Halpern EM, Lovblom LE, Weisman A, Orlov S, Bril V, Perkins BA. Structure-function relationship between corneal nerves and conventional small-fiber tests in type 1 diabetes. Diabetes Care. 2013 Sep 1;36(9):2748-55.

Taylor SI, Blau JE, Rother KI. SGLT2 Inhibitors May Predispose to Ketoacidosis. J Clin Endocrinol Metab. 2015 Aug;100(8):2849-52. doi: 10.1210/jc.2015-1884. Epub 2015 Jun 18. PMID: 26086329; PMCID: PMC4525004.

Weinstock RS, Xing D, Maahs DM, Michels A, Rickels MR, Peters AL, Bergenstal RM, Harris B, Dubose SN, Miller KM, Beck RW; T1D Exchange Clinic Network. Severe hypoglycemia and diabetic ketoacidosis in adults with type 1 diabetes: results from the T1D Exchange clinic registry. J Clin Endocrinol Metab. 2013 Aug;98(8):3411-9. doi: 10.1210/jc.2013-1589. Epub 2013 Jun 12. PMID: 23760624.

Weisman A, Lovblom LE, Keenan HA, Tinsley LJ, D'Eon S, Boulet G, Farooqi MA, Lovshin JA, Orszag A, Lytvyn Y, Brent MH, Paul N, Bril V, Cherney DZ, Perkins BA. Diabetes Care Disparities in Long-standing Type 1 Diabetes in Canada and the U.S.: A Cross-sectional Comparison. Diabetes Care. 2018 Jan;41(1):88-95. doi: 10.2337/dc17-1074. Epub 2017 Nov 8. PMID: 29118059; PMCID: PMC5741151.

Zinman B, Wanner C, Lachin JM, Fitchett D, Bluhmki E, Hantel S, Mattheus M, Devins T, Johansen OE, Woerle HJ, Broedl UC, Inzucchi SE; EMPA-REG OUTCOME Investigators. Empagliflozin, Cardiovascular Outcomes, and Mortality in Type 2 Diabetes. N Engl J Med. 2015 Nov 26;373(22):2117-28. doi: 10.1056/NEJMoa1504720. Epub 2015 Sep 17. PMID: 26378978.

Chapter Four

Brennan DC, Kopetskie HA, Sayre PH, Alejandro R, Cagliero E, Shapiro AM, Goldstein JS, DesMarais MR, Booher S, Bianchine PJ. Long-Term Follow-Up of the Edmonton Protocol of Islet Transplantation in the United States. Am J Transplant. 2016 Feb;16(2):509-17. doi: 10.1111/ajt.13458. Epub 2015 Oct 3. PMID: 26433206.

Lakey JRT, Rajotte RV, Fedorow CA, Taylor MJ. Islet Cryopreservation Using Intracellular Preservation Solutions. Cell Transplantation. October 2001:583-589. doi:10.3727/000000001783986369

Neitz, Ross. Edmonton Protocol: The past, present and bright future of a diabetes breakthrough. Folio, November 14, 2016.

Pepper AR, Bruni A, Shapiro AMJ. Clinical islet transplantation: is the future finally now? Curr Opin Organ Transplant. 2018 Aug;23(4):428-439. doi: 10.1097/MOT.0000000000000546. PMID: 29847441.

Rajotte RV. Islet cryopreservation protocols. Ann N Y Acad Sci. 1999 Jun 18;875:200-7. doi: 10.1111/j.1749-6632.1999.tb08504.x. PMID: 10415568.

Rajotte RV. Cryopreservation of pancreatic islets. Transplant Proc. 1994 Apr;26(2):395-6. PMID: 8171474.

Rajotte RV, Evans MG, Warnock GL, Kneteman NM. Islet cryopreservation. Horm Metab Res Suppl. 1990;25:72-81. PMID: 2088990.

Shapiro AM, Lakey JR, Ryan EA, Korbutt GS, Toth E, Warnock GL, Kneteman NM, Rajotte RV. Islet transplantation in seven patients with type 1 diabetes mellitus using a glucocorticoid-free immunosuppressive regimen. N Engl J Med. 2000 Jul 27;343(4):230-8. doi: 10.1056/NEJM200007273430401. PMID: 10911004.

Shapiro AM, Ricordi C, Hering BJ, Auchincloss H, Lindblad R, Robertson RP, Secchi A, Brendel MD, Berney T, Brennan DC, Cagliero E, Alejandro R, Ryan EA, DiMercurio B, Morel P, Polonsky KS, Reems JA, Bretzel RG, Bertuzzi F, Froud T, Kandaswamy R, Sutherland DE, Eisenbarth G, Segal M, Preiksaitis J, Korbutt GS, Barton FB, Viviano L, Seyfert-Margolis V, Bluestone J, Lakey JR. International trial of the Edmonton protocol for islet transplantation. N Engl J Med. 2006 Sep 28;355(13):1318-30. doi: 10.1056/NEJMoa061267. PMID: 17005949.

Chapter Five

Aghazadeh Y, Nostro MC. Cell Therapy for Type 1 Diabetes: Current and Future Strategies. Curr Diab Rep. 2017 Jun;17(6):37. doi: 10.1007/s11892-017-0863-6. PMID: 28432571.

Cogger K, Nostro MC. Recent advances in cell replacement therapies for the treatment of type 1 diabetes. Endocrinology. 2015 Jan;156(1):8-15. doi: 10.1210/en.2014-1691. PMID: 25386833.

Gamble A, Pepper AR, Bruni A, Shapiro AMJ. The journey of islet cell transplantation and future development. Islets. 2018 Mar 4;10(2):80-94. doi: 10.1080/19382014.2018.1428511. Epub 2018 Feb 5. PMID: 29394145; PMCID: PMC5895174.

Kieffer TJ. Closing in on Mass Production of Mature Human Beta Cells. Cell Stem Cell. 2016 Jun 2;18(6):699-702. doi: 10.1016/j.stem.2016.05.014. PMID: 27257758.

Lyon J, Manning Fox JE, Spigelman AF, Kim R, Smith N, O'Gorman D, Kin T, Shapiro AM, Rajotte RV, MacDonald PE. Research-Focused Isolation of Human Islets From Donors With and Without Diabetes at the Alberta Diabetes Institute IsletCore. Endocrinology. 2016 Feb;157(2):560-9. doi: 10.1210/en.2015-1562. Epub 2015 Dec 11. PMID: 26653569.

McCulloch EA, Till, The radiation sensitivity of normal mouse bone marrow cells, determined by quantitative marrow transplantation into irradiated mice. Radiat Res. 1960 Jul;13:115-25. PMID: 13858509.

Nostro MC, Cheng X, Keller GM, Gadue P. Wnt, activin, and BMP signaling regulate distinct stages in the developmental pathway from embryonic stem cells to blood. Cell Stem Cell. 2008 Jan 10;2(1):60-71. doi: 10.1016/j.stem.2007.10.011. PMID: 18371422; PMCID: PMC2533280.

Nostro MC, Sarangi F, Ogawa S, Holtzinger A, Corneo B, Li X, Micallef SJ, Park IH, Basford C, Wheeler MB, Daley GQ, Elefanty AG, Stanley EG, Keller G. Stage-specific signaling through TGFβ family members and WNT regulates patterning and pancreatic specification of human pluripotent stem cells. Development. 2011 Mar;138(5):861-71. doi: 10.1242/dev.055236. Epub 2011 Jan 26. Erratum in: Development. 2011 Apr;138(7):1445. Erratum in: Development. 2011 Mar;138(5).doi: 10.1242/dev.065904. PMID: 21270052; PMCID: PMC3035090.

Nostro MC, Sarangi F, Yang C, Holland A, Elefanty AG, Stanley EG, Greiner DL, Keller G. Efficient generation of NKX6-1+ pancreatic progenitors from multiple human pluripotent stem cell lines. Stem Cell Reports. 2015 Apr 14;4(4):591-604. doi: 10.1016/j.stemcr.2015.02.017. Epub 2015 Apr 2. PMID: 25843049; PMCID: PMC4400642.

Rezania A, Bruin JE, Arora P, Rubin A, Batushansky I, Asadi A, O'Dwyer S, Quiskamp N, Mojibian M, Albrecht T, Yang YH, Johnson JD, Kieffer TJ. Reversal of diabetes with insulin-producing cells derived in vitro from human pluripotent stem cells. Nat Biotechnol. 2014 Nov;32(11):1121-33. doi: 10.1038/nbt.3033. Epub 2014 Sep 11. PMID: 25211370.

Shore, Randy. Stem cell implant trial aims to reverse Type 1 diabetes. Vancouver Sun, January 16, 2018.

Till JE, McCulloch EA, A direct measurement of the radiation sensitivity of normal mouse bone marrow cells. Radiat Res. 1961 Feb;14:213-22. PMID: 13776896.

Willemse, Lisa. U of T researchers tackle type 1 diabetes with regenerative medicine technologies. U of T News, July 10, 2018

Chapter Six

Bruin JE, Kellenberger LD, Gerstein HC, Morrison KM, Holloway AC. Fetal and neonatal nicotine exposure and postnatal glucose homeostasis: identifying critical windows of exposure. J Endocrinol. 2007;194(1):171-178. doi:10.1677/JOE-07-0050

Bruin JE, Petre MA, Lehman MA, et al. Maternal nicotine exposure increases oxidative stress in the offspring. Free Radic Biol Med. 2008;44(11):1919-1925. doi:10.1016/j.freeradbiomed.2008.02.010

Bruin JE, Gerstein HC, Holloway AC. Long-term consequences of fetal and neonatal nicotine exposure: a critical review. Toxicol Sci. 2010;116(2):364-374. doi:10.1093/toxsci/kfq103

Bruin JE, Rezania A, Xu J, et al. Maturation and function of human embryonic stem cell-derived pancreatic progenitors in macroencapsulation devices following transplant into mice. Diabetologia. 2013;56(9):1987-1998. doi:10.1007/s00125-013-2955-4

Bruin JE, Erener S, Vela J, et al. Characterization of polyhormonal insulin-producing cells derived in vitro from human embryonic stem cells. Stem Cell Res. 2014;12(1):194-208. doi:10.1016/j.scr.2013.10.003

Johnson JD. The quest to make fully functional human pancreatic beta cells from embryonic stem cells: climbing a mountain in the clouds. Diabetologia. 2016;59(10):2047-2057. doi:10.1007/s00125-016-4059-4

Johnson JD, Luciani DS. Mechanisms of pancreatic beta-cell apoptosis in diabetes and its therapies. Adv Exp Med Biol. 2010;654:447-462. doi:10.1007/978-90-481-3271-3_19

Rezania A, Bruin JE, Arora P, et al. Reversal of diabetes with insulin-producing cells derived in vitro from human pluripotent stem cells. Nat Biotechnol. 2014;32(11):1121-1133. doi:10.1038/nbt.3033

Rezania A, Bruin JE, Riedel MJ, et al. Maturation of human embryonic stem cell-derived pancreatic progenitors into functional islets capable of treating pre-existing diabetes in mice. *Diabetes.* 2012;61(8):2016-2029. doi:10.2337/db11-1711.

Rezania A, Bruin JE, Xu J, et al. Enrichment of human embryonic stem cell-derived NKX6.1-expressing pancreatic progenitor cells accelerates the maturation of insulin-secreting cells in vivo. *Stem Cells.* 2013;31(11):2432-2442. doi:10.1002/stem.1489.

Templeman NM, Clee SM, Johnson JD. Suppression of hyperinsulinaemia in growing female mice provides long-term protection against obesity. *Diabetologia.* 2015;58(10):2392-2402. doi:10.1007/s00125-015-3676-7.

Interlude: Dr. Derek van der Kooy

Arntfield ME, van der Kooy D. β-Cell evolution: How the pancreas borrowed from the brain: The shared toolbox of genes expressed by neural and pancreatic endocrine cells may reflect their evolutionary relationship. Bioessays. 2011 Aug;33(8):582-7. doi: 10.1002/bies.201100015. Epub 2011 Jun 16. PMID: 21681773.

Seaberg RM, Smukler SR, Kieffer TJ, Enikolopov G, Asghar Z, Wheeler MB, Korbutt G, van der Kooy D. Clonal identification of multipotent precursors from adult mouse pancreas that generate neural and pancreatic lineages. Nat Biotechnol. 2004 Sep;22(9):1115-24. doi: 10.1038/nbt1004. Epub 2004 Aug 22. PMID: 15322557.

Smukler SR, Arntfield ME, Razavi R, Bikopoulos G, Karpowicz P, Seaberg R, Dai F, Lee S, Ahrens R, Fraser PE, Wheeler MB, van der Kooy D. The adult mouse and human pancreas contain rare multipotent stem cells that express insulin. Cell Stem Cell. 2011 Mar 4;8(3):281-93. doi: 10.1016/j.stem.2011.01.015. PMID: 21362568.

Chapter Seven

Costa M, Potvin S, Berthiaume Y, Gauthier L, Jeanneret A, Lavoie A, Levesque R, Chiasson J, Rabasa-Lhoret R. Diabetes: a major co-morbidity of cystic fibrosis. Diabetes Metab. 2005 Jun;31(3 Pt 1):221-32. doi: 10.1016/s1262-3636(07)70189-1. PMID: 16142013.

Haidar A, Legault L, Dallaire M, Alkhateeb A, Coriati A, Messier V, Cheng P, Millette M, Boulet B, Rabasa-Lhoret R. Glucose-responsive insulin and glucagon delivery (dual-hormone artificial pancreas) in adults with type 1 diabetes: a randomized crossover controlled trial. CMAJ. 2013 Mar 5;185(4):297-305. doi: 10.1503/cmaj.121265. Epub 2013 Jan 28. PMID: 23359039; PMCID: PMC3589308.

Haidar A, Legault L, Matteau-Pelletier L, Messier V, Dallaire M, Ladouceur M, Rabasa-Lhoret R. Outpatient overnight glucose control with dual-hormone artificial pancreas, single-hormone artificial pancreas, or conventional insulin pump therapy in children and adolescents with type 1 diabetes: an open-label, randomised controlled trial. Lancet Diabetes Endocrinol. 2015 Aug;3(8):595-604. doi: 10.1016/S2213-8587(15)00141-2. Epub 2015 Jun 8. PMID: 26066705.

Haidar A, Legault L, Messier V, Mitre TM, Leroux C, Rabasa-Lhoret R. Comparison of dual-hormone artificial pancreas, single-hormone artificial pancreas, and conventional insulin pump therapy for glycaemic control in patients with type 1 diabetes: an open-label randomised controlled crossover trial. Lancet Diabetes Endocrinol. 2015 Jan;3(1):17-26. doi: 10.1016/S2213-8587(14)70226-8. Epub 2014 Nov 27. PMID: 25434967.

Haidar A, Rabasa-Lhoret R, Legault L, Lovblom LE, Rakheja R, Messier V, D'Aoust É, Falappa CM, Justice T, Orszag A, Tschirhart H, Dallaire M, Ladouceur M, Perkins BA. Single- and Dual-Hormone Artificial Pancreas for Overnight Glucose Control in Type 1 Diabetes. J Clin Endocrinol Metab. 2016 Jan;101(1):214-23. doi: 10.1210/jc.2015-3003. Epub 2015 Nov 2. PMID: 26523526.

Haidar A, Tsoukas MA, Bernier-Twardy S, Yale JF, Rutkowski J, Bossy A, Pytka E, El Fathi A, Strauss N, Legault L. A Novel Dual-Hormone Insulin-and-Pramlintide Artificial Pancreas for Type 1 Diabetes: A Randomized Controlled Crossover Trial. Diabetes Care. 2020 Mar;43(3):597-606. doi: 10.2337/dc19-1922. Epub 2020 Jan 23. PMID: 31974099.

Ohlendorf, Pat. New Assaults on Diabetes. Maclean's Magazine, May 18, 1981.

Perkins BA, Cardinez N, Opsteen CF. Talking Points for Helping Your Type 1 Diabetes Patient Decide About Hybrid Closed Loop. Can J Diabetes. 2020 Jun;44(4):356-358. doi: 10.1016/j.jcjd.2019.10.004. Epub 2019 Oct 26. PMID: 31866241.

Chapter Eight

Diabetes Canada Clinical Practice Guidelines Expert Committee, Feig DS, Berger H, Donovan L, Godbout A, Kader T, Keely E, Sanghera R. Diabetes and Pregnancy. Can J Diabetes. 2018 Apr;42 Suppl 1:S255-S282. doi: 10.1016/j.jcjd.2017.10.038. Erratum in: Can J Diabetes. 2018 Jun;42(3):337. PMID: 29650105.

Feig DS, Donovan LE, Corcoy R, Murphy KE, Amiel SA, Hunt KF, Asztalos E, Barrett JFR, Sanchez JJ, de Leiva A, Hod M, Jovanovic L, Keely E, McManus R, Hutton EK, Meek CL, Stewart ZA, Wysocki T, O'Brien R, Ruedy K, Kollman C, Tomlinson G, Murphy HR; CONCEPTT Collaborative Group. Continuous glucose monitoring in pregnant women with type 1 diabetes (CONCEPTT): a multicentre international randomised controlled trial. Lancet. 2017 Nov 25;390(10110):2347-2359. doi: 10.1016/S0140-6736(17)32400-5. Epub 2017 Sep 15. Erratum in: Lancet. 2017 Nov 25;390(10110):2346. PMID: 28923465; PMCID: PMC5713979.

Feig DS, Murphy HR. Continuous glucose monitoring in pregnant women with Type 1 diabetes: benefits for mothers, using pumps or pens, and their babies. Diabet Med. 2018 Apr;35(4):430-435. doi: 10.1111/dme.13585. Epub 2018 Feb 15. PMID: 29352491.

Joham AE, Ranasinha S, Zoungas S, Moran L, Teede HJ. Gestational diabetes and type 2 diabetes in reproductive-aged women with polycystic ovary syndrome. J Clin Endocrinol Metab. 2014 Mar;99(3):E447-52. doi: 10.1210/jc.2013-2007. Epub 2013 Sep 30. PMID: 24081730.

Kew S, Ye C, Sermer M, Connelly PW, Hanley AJ, Zinman B, Retnakaran R. Postpartum metabolic function in women delivering a macrosomic infant in the absence of gestational diabetes mellitus. Diabetes Care. 2011 Dec;34(12):2608-13. doi: 10.2337/dc11-1554. Epub 2011 Oct 4. PMID: 21972414; PMCID: PMC3220842.

Lega IC, Wilton AS, Austin PC, Fischer HD, Johnson JA, Lipscombe LL. The temporal relationship between diabetes and cancer: A population-based study. Cancer. 2016 Sep 1;122(17):2731-8. doi: 10.1002/cncr.30095. Epub 2016 Jul 11. PMID: 27400035.

Lipscombe LL, Hux JE, Booth GL. Reduced screening mammography among women with diabetes. Arch Intern Med. 2005 Oct 10;165(18):2090-5. doi: 10.1001/archinte.165.18.2090. PMID: 16216998.

Lipscombe LL, McLaughlin HM, Wu W, Feig DS. Pregnancy planning in women with pregestational diabetes. J Matern Fetal Neonatal Med. 2011 Sep;24(9):1095-101. doi: 10.3109/14767058.2010.545929. Epub 2011 Jan 24. PMID: 21261446.

Lipscombe LL, Goodwin PJ, Zinman B, McLaughlin JR, Hux JE. Diabetes mellitus and breast cancer: a retrospective population-based cohort study. Breast Cancer Res Treat. 2006 Aug;98(3):349-56. doi: 10.1007/s10549-006-9172-5. Epub 2006 Mar 16. PMID: 16541321.

Lipscombe LL, Fischer HD, Austin PC, Fu L, Jaakkimainen RL, Ginsburg O, Rochon PA, Narod S, Paszat L. The association between diabetes and breast cancer stage at diagnosis: a population-based study. Breast Cancer Res Treat. 2015 Apr;150(3):613-20. doi: 10.1007/s10549-015-3323-5. Epub 2015 Mar 17. PMID: 25779100.

Lipscombe LL, Delos-Reyes F, Glenn AJ, de Sequeira S, Liang X, Grant S, Thorpe KE, Price JAD. The Avoiding Diabetes After Pregnancy Trial in Moms Program: Feasibility of a Diabetes Prevention Program for Women With Recent Gestational Diabetes Mellitus. Can J Diabetes. 2019 Dec;43(8):613-620. doi: 10.1016/j.jcjd.2019.08.019. Epub 2019 Sep 25. PMID: 31669188.

Peticca P, Shah BR, Shea A, Clark HD, Malcolm JC, Walker M, Karovitch A, Brazeau-Gravelle P, Keely EJ. Clinical predictors for diabetes screening in the first year postpartum after gestational diabetes. Obstet Med. 2014 Sep;7(3):116-20. doi: 10.1177/1753495X14528487. Epub 2014 Apr 14. PMID: 27512435; PMCID: PMC4934972.

Retnakaran R, Hanley AJ, Raif N, Connelly PW, Sermer M, Zinman B. Reduced adiponectin concentration in women with gestational diabetes: a potential factor in progression to type 2 diabetes. Diabetes Care. 2004 Mar;27(3):799-800. doi: 10.2337/diacare.27.3.799. PMID: 14988306.

Retnakaran R, Hanley AJ, Raif N, Hirning CR, Connelly PW, Sermer M, Kahn SE, Zinman B. Adiponectin and beta cell dysfunction in gestational diabetes: pathophysiological implications. Diabetologia. 2005 May;48(5):993-1001. doi: 10.1007/s00125-005-1710-x. Epub 2005 Mar 19. PMID: 15778860.

Retnakaran R, Zinman B, Connelly PW, Sermer M, Hanley AJ. Impaired glucose tolerance of pregnancy is a heterogeneous metabolic disorder as defined by the glycemic response to the oral glucose tolerance test. Diabetes Care. 2006 Jan;29(1):57-62. doi: 10.2337/diacare.29.1.57. PMID: 16373896.

Shah BR, Lipscombe LL, Feig DS, Lowe JM. Missed opportunities for type 2 diabetes testing following gestational diabetes: a population-based cohort study. BJOG. 2011 Nov;118(12):1484-90. doi: 10.1111/j.1471-0528.2011.03083.x. Epub 2011 Aug 22. PMID: 21864326.

Chapter Nine

Blotsky AL, Rahme E, Dahhou M, Nakhla M, Dasgupta K. Gestational diabetes associated with incident diabetes in childhood and youth: a retrospective cohort study. CMAJ. 2019 Apr 15;191(15):E410-E417. doi: 10.1503/cmaj.181001. PMID: 30988041; PMCID: PMC6464886.

Brazeau AS, Nakhla M, Wright M, Henderson M, Panagiotopoulos C, Pacaud D, Kearns P, Rahme E, Da Costa D, Dasgupta K. Stigma and Its Association With Glycemic Control and Hypoglycemia in Adolescents and Young Adults With Type 1 Diabetes: Cross-Sectional Study. J Med Internet Res. 2018 Apr 20;20(4):e151. doi: 10.2196/jmir.9432. PMID: 29678801; PMCID: PMC5935805.

Brazeau, A., Meltzer, S.J., Pace, R. et al. Health behaviour changes in partners of women with recent gestational diabetes: a phase IIa trial. BMC Public Health 18, 575 (2018). https://doi.org/10.1186/s12889-018-5490-x

Dasgupta K, Rosenberg E, Joseph L, Cooke AB, Trudeau L, Bacon SL, Chan D, Sherman M, Rabasa-Lhoret R, Daskalopoulou SS; SMARTER Trial Group. Physician step prescription and monitoring to improve ARTERial health (SMARTER): A randomized controlled trial in patients with type 2 diabetes and hypertension. Diabetes Obes Metab. 2017 May;19(5):695-704. doi: 10.1111/dom.12874. Epub 2017 Feb 22. PMID: 28074635; PMCID: PMC5412851.

Dasgupta K, Ross N, Meltzer S, Da Costa D, Nakhla M, Habel Y, Rahme E. Gestational Diabetes Mellitus in Mothers as a Diabetes Predictor in Fathers: A Retrospective Cohort Analysis. Diabetes Care. 2015 Sep;38(9):e130-1. doi: 10.2337/dc15-0855. Epub 2015 Jun 26. PMID: 26116719.

Leong A, Rahme E, Dasgupta K. Spousal diabetes as a diabetes risk factor: a systematic review and meta-analysis. BMC Med. 2014 Jan 24;12:12. doi: 10.1186/1741-7015-12-12. PMID: 24460622; PMCID: PMC3900990.

Leong A, Dasgupta K, Chiasson JL, Rahme E. Estimating the population prevalence of diagnosed and undiagnosed diabetes. Diabetes Care. 2013 Oct;36(10):3002-8. doi: 10.2337/dc12-2543. Epub 2013 May 8. PMID: 23656982; PMCID: PMC3781536.

Pace R, Brazeau AS, Meltzer S, Rahme E, Dasgupta K. Conjoint Associations of Gestational Diabetes and Hypertension With Diabetes, Hypertension, and Cardiovascular Disease in Parents: A Retrospective Cohort Study. Am J Epidemiol. 2017 Nov 15;186(10):1115-1124. doi: 10.1093/aje/kwx263. PMID: 29149255; PMCID: PMC5859985.

Chapter Ten

Creatore MI, Glazier RH, Moineddin R, Fazli GS, Johns A, Gozdyra P, Matheson FI, Kaufman-Shriqui V, Rosella LC, Manuel DG, Booth GL. Association of Neighborhood Walkability With Change in Overweight, Obesity, and Diabetes. JAMA. 2016 May 24-31;315(20):2211-20. doi: 10.1001/jama.2016.5898. PMID: 27218630.

Booth GL, Creatore MI, Moineddin R, Gozdyra P, Weyman JT, Matheson FI, Glazier RH. Unwalkable neighborhoods, poverty, and the risk of diabetes among recent immigrants to Canada compared with long-term residents. Diabetes Care. 2013 Feb;36(2):302-8. doi: 10.2337/dc12-0777. Epub 2012 Sep 17. PMID: 22988302; PMCID: PMC3554289.

Booth GL, Creatore MI, Luo J, Fazli GS, Johns A, Rosella LC, Glazier RH, Moineddin R, Gozdyra P, Austin PC. Neighbourhood walkability and the incidence of diabetes: an inverse probability of treatment weighting analysis. J Epidemiol

Community Health. 2019 Apr;73(4):287-294. doi: 10.1136/jech-2018-210510. Epub 2019 Jan 29. PMID: 30696690.

Fazli GS, Moineddin R, Chu A, Bierman AS, Booth GL. Neighborhood walkability and pre-diabetes incidence in a multiethnic population. BMJ Open Diabetes Res Care. 2020 Jun;8(1):e000908. doi: 10.1136/bmjdrc-2019-000908. PMID: 32601153; PMCID: PMC7326269.

Howell NA, Tu JV, Moineddin R, Chen H, Chu A, Hystad P, Booth GL. Interaction between neighborhood walkability and traffic-related air pollution on hypertension and diabetes: The CANHEART cohort. Environ Int. 2019 Nov;132:104799. doi: 10.1016/j.envint.2019.04.070. Epub 2019 Jun 25. PMID: 31253484.

Howell NA, Tu JV, Moineddin R, Chen H, Chu A, Hystad P, Booth GL. The probability of diabetes and hypertension by levels of neighborhood walkability and traffic-related air pollution across 15 municipalities in Southern Ontario, Canada: A dataset derived from 2,496,458 community dwelling-adults. Data Brief. 2019 Aug 28;27:104439. doi: 10.1016/j.dib.2019.104439. PMID: 31720317; PMCID: PMC6838449.

Hux JE, Ivis F, Flintoft V, Bica A. Diabetes in Ontario: determination of prevalence and incidence using a validated administrative data algorithm. Diabetes Care. 2002 Mar;25(3):512-6. doi: 10.2337/diacare.25.3.512. PMID: 11874939.

ICES. Fast-food "swamps" linked to high rates of obesity, when healthier choices crowded out: Ontario study. ICES website, December 1, 2015.

Lipscombe LL, Hux JE. Trends in diabetes prevalence, incidence, and mortality in Ontario, Canada 1995-2005: a population-based study. Lancet. 2007 Mar 3;369(9563):750-756. doi: 10.1016/S0140-6736(07)60361-4. PMID: 17336651.

Lipscombe LL, Austin PC, Manuel DG, Shah BR, Hux JE, Booth GL. Income-related differences in mortality among people with diabetes mellitus. CMAJ. 2010 Jan 12;182(1):E1-E17. doi: 10.1503/cmaj.090495. Epub 2009 Dec 21. PMID: 20026629; PMCID: PMC2802626.

Polsky JY, Moineddin R, Glazier RH, Dunn JR, Booth GL. Foodscapes of southern Ontario: neighbourhood deprivation and access to healthy and unhealthy food retail. Can J Public Health. 2014 Jul 31;105(5):e369-75. doi: 10.17269/cjph.105.4541. PMID: 25365272; PMCID: PMC6972074.

Polsky JY, Moineddin R, Dunn JR, Glazier RH, Booth GL. Absolute and relative densities of fast-food versus other restaurants in relation to weight status: Does restaurant mix matter? Prev Med. 2016 Jan;82:28-34. doi: 10.1016/j.ypmed.2015.11.008. Epub 2015 Nov 12. PMID: 26582211.

Weisman A, Tu K, Young J, Kumar M, Austin PC, Jaakkimainen L, Lipscombe L, Aronson R, Booth GL. Validation of a type 1 diabetes algorithm using electronic medical records and administrative healthcare data to study the population incidence and prevalence of type 1 diabetes in Ontario, Canada. BMJ Open Diabetes Res Care. 2020 Jun;8(1):e001224. doi: 10.1136/bmjdrc-2020-001224. PMID: 32565422; PMCID: PMC7307536.

Interlude: Dr. David Campbell

Campbell DJ, Gibson K, O'Neill BG, Thurston WE. The role of a student-run clinic in providing primary care for Calgary's homeless populations: a qualitative study. BMC Health Serv Res. 2013 Jul 17;13:277. doi: 10.1186/1472-6963-13-277. PMID: 23866968; PMCID: PMC3718696.

Campbell DJT, Campbell RB, Ziegler C, Mcbrien KA, Hwang SW, Booth GL. Interventions for improved diabetes control and self-management among those experiencing homelessness: protocol for a mixed methods scoping review. Syst Rev. 2019 Apr 22;8(1):100. doi: 10.1186/s13643-019-1020-x. PMID: 31010419; PMCID: PMC6477731

Campbell DJT, Campbell RB, Booth GL, Hwang SW, McBrien KA. Innovations in Providing Diabetes Care for Individuals Experiencing Homelessness: An Environmental Scan. Can J Diabetes. 2020 Oct;44(7):643-650. doi: 10.1016/j. jcjd.2020.01.011. Epub 2020 Feb 14. PMID: 32312657.

Chapter Eleven

Jones A, Vallis M, Pouwer F. If it does not significantly change HbA1c levels why should we waste time on it? A plea for the prioritization of psychological well-being in people with diabetes. Diabet Med. 2015 Feb;32(2):155-63. doi: 10.1111/dme.12620. Epub 2014 Dec 10. PMID: 25354315.

Jones A, Vallis M, Cooke D, Pouwer F. Working Together to Promote Diabetes Control: A Practical Guide for Diabetes Health Care Providers in Establishing a Working Alliance to Achieve Self-Management Support. J Diabetes Res. 2016;2016:2830910. doi: 10.1155/2016/2830910. Epub 2015 Nov 22. PMID: 26682229; PMCID: PMC4670648.

Nichols J, Vallis M, Boutette S, Gall Casey C, Yu CH. A Canadian Cross-Sectional Survey on Psychosocial Supports for Adults Living With Type 1 or 2 Diabetes: Health-Care Providers' Awareness, Capacity and Motivation. Can J Diabetes. 2018 Aug;42(4):389-394.e2. doi: 10.1016/j.jcjd.2017.09.004. Epub 2017 Nov 9. PMID: 29129456.

Nicolucci A, Kovacs Burns K, Holt RI, Comaschi M, Hermanns N, Ishii H, Kokoszka A, Pouwer F, Skovlund SE, Stuckey H, Tarkun I, Vallis M, Wens J, Peyrot M; DAWN2 Study Group. Diabetes Attitudes, Wishes and Needs second study (DAWN2™): cross-national benchmarking of diabetes-related psychosocial outcomes for people with diabetes. Diabet Med. 2013 Jul;30(7):767-77. doi: 10.1111/dme.12245. Erratum in: Diabet Med. 2013 Oct;30(10):1266. PMID: 23711019.

Peyrot M, Rubin RR, Lauritzen T, Snoek FJ, Matthews DR, Skovlund SE. Psychosocial problems and barriers to improved diabetes management: results of the Cross-National Diabetes Attitudes, Wishes and Needs (DAWN) Study. Diabet Med. 2005 Oct;22(10):1379-85. doi: 10.1111/j.1464-5491.2005.01644.x. PMID: 16176200.

Stenov V, Wind G, Vallis M, Reventlow S, Hempler NF. Group-based, person-centered diabetes self-management education: healthcare professionals' implementation of new approaches. BMC Health Serv Res. 2019 Jun 11;19(1):368. doi: 10.1186/s12913-019-4183-1. PMID: 31185968; PMCID: PMC6558764.

Stuckey HL, Vallis M, Kovacs Burns K, Mullan-Jensen CB, Reading JM, Kalra S, Wens J, Kokoszka A, Skovlund SE, Peyrot M. "I Do My Best To Listen to Patients": Qualitative Insights Into DAWN2 (Diabetes Psychosocial Care From the Perspective of Health Care Professionals in the Second Diabetes Attitudes, Wishes and Needs Study). Clin Ther. 2015 Sep;37(9):1986-1998.e12. doi: 10.1016/j.clinthera.2015.06.010. Epub 2015 Jul 10. PMID: 26169765.

Vallis M, Jones A, Pouwer F. Managing hypoglycemia in diabetes may be more fear management than glucose management: a practical guide for diabetes care providers. Curr Diabetes Rev. 2014;10(6):364-70. doi: 10.2174/1573399810666 141113115026. PMID: 25394991.

Chapter Twelve

Aronson R, Brown RE, Li A, Riddell MC. Optimal Insulin Correction Factor in Post-High-Intensity Exercise Hyperglycemia in Adults With Type 1 Diabetes: The FIT Study. Diabetes Care. 2019 Jan;42(1):10-16. doi: 10.2337/dc18-1475. Epub 2018 Nov 19. PMID: 30455336.

Colberg SR, Sigal RJ, Yardley JE, Riddell MC, Dunstan DW, Dempsey PC, Horton ES, Castorino K, Tate DF. Physical Activity/Exercise and Diabetes: A Position Statement of the American Diabetes Association. Diabetes Care. 2016 Nov;39(11):2065-2079. doi: 10.2337/dc16-1728. PMID: 27926890; PMCID: PMC6908414.

Iqbal, Maria. Dogged researcher helped advance the understanding of diabetes. The Globe and Mail, July 17, 2019

Jendle JH, Riddell MC. Editorial: Physical Activity and Type 1 Diabetes. Front Endocrinol (Lausanne). 2019 Dec 6;10:860. doi: 10.3389/fendo.2019.00860. PMID: 31866952; PMCID: PMC6908475.

Scott SN, Christiansen MP, Fontana FY, Stettler C, Bracken RM, Hayes CA, Fisher M, Bode B, Lagrou PH, Southerland P, Riddell MC. Evaluation of Factors Related to Glycemic Management in Professional Cyclists With Type 1 Diabetes Over a 7-Day Stage Race. Diabetes Care. 2020 May;43(5):1142-1145. doi: 10.2337/dc19-2302. Epub 2020 Mar 16. PMID: 32179510; PMCID: PMC7171953.

Rickels MR, DuBose SN, Toschi E, Beck RW, Verdejo AS, Wolpert H, Cummins MJ, Newswanger B, Riddell MC; T1D Exchange Mini-Dose Glucagon Exercise Study Group. Mini-Dose Glucagon as a Novel Approach to Prevent Exercise-Induced Hypoglycemia in Type 1 Diabetes. Diabetes Care. 2018 Sep;41(9):1909-1916. doi: 10.2337/dc18-0051. Epub 2018 May 18. PMID: 29776987; PMCID: PMC6463733.

Riddell MC, Zaharieva DP, Yavelberg L, Cinar A, Jamnik VK. Exercise and the Development of the Artificial Pancreas: One of the More Difficult Series of Hurdles. J Diabetes Sci Technol. 2015 Oct 1;9(6):1217-26. doi: 10.1177/1932296815609370. PMID: 26428933; PMCID: PMC4667314.

Riddell MC, Gallen IW, Smart CE, Taplin CE, Adolfsson P, Lumb AN, Kowalski A, Rabasa-Lhoret R, McCrimmon RJ, Hume C, Annan F, Fournier PA, Graham C, Bode B, Galassetti P, Jones TW, Millán IS, Heise T, Peters AL, Petz A, Laffel LM. Exercise management in type 1 diabetes: a consensus statement. Lancet Diabetes Endocrinol. 2017 May;5(5):377-390. doi: 10.1016/S2213-8587(17)30014-1. Epub 2017 Jan 24. Erratum in: Lancet Diabetes Endocrinol. 2017 May;5(5):e3. PMID: 28126459.

Riddell MC, Zaharieva DP, Tansey M, Tsalikian E, Admon G, Li Z, Kollman C, Beck RW. Individual glucose responses to prolonged moderate intensity aerobic exercise in adolescents with type 1 diabetes: The higher they start, the harder they fall. Pediatr Diabetes. 2019 Feb;20(1):99-106. doi: 10.1111/pedi.12799. Epub 2018 Dec 13. PMID: 30467929.

Zaharieva DP, Riddell MC, Henske J. The Accuracy of Continuous Glucose Monitoring and Flash Glucose Monitoring During Aerobic Exercise in Type 1 Diabetes. J Diabetes Sci Technol. 2019 Jan;13(1):140-141. doi: 10.1177/1932296818804550. Epub 2018 Oct 7. PMID: 30295040; PMCID: PMC6313274.

Zaharieva DP, Turksoy K, McGaugh SM, Pooni R, Vienneau T, Ly T, Riddell MC. Lag Time Remains with Newer Real-Time Continuous Glucose Monitoring Technology During Aerobic Exercise in Adults Living with Type 1 Diabetes. Diabetes Technol Ther. 2019 Jun;21(6):313-321. doi: 10.1089/dia.2018.0364. Epub 2019 May 6. PMID: 31059282; PMCID: PMC6551983.

Zaharieva DP, Cinar A, Yavelberg L, Jamnik V, Riddell MC. No Disadvantage to Insulin Pump Off vs Pump On During Intermittent High-Intensity Exercise in Adults With Type 1 Diabetes. Can J Diabetes. 2020 Mar;44(2):162-168. doi: 10.1016/j.jcjd.2019.05.015. Epub 2019 Jun 7. PMID: 31416695.

Index

About the Author

Krista Lamb is a Toronto-based writer, podcast producer and host. She specializes in turning complex medical science into compelling stories that will help listeners and readers understand why this science truly matters in their lives. She is passionate about the role of research in establishing new treatments and, one day, a cure for diabetes.

You can find more of her work and sign up for her newsletter at kristalamb.com.

CPSIA information can be obtained
at www.ICGtesting.com
Printed in the USA
BVHW080044041121
620619BV00008B/139